Pneumonia

Edited by Nima Rezaei

Published in London, United Kingdom

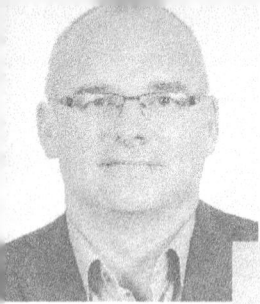
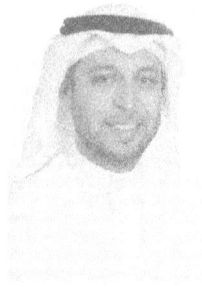
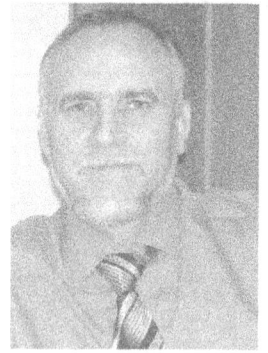
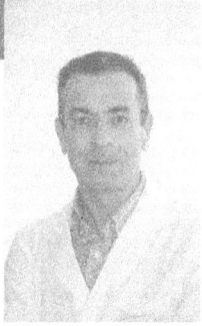
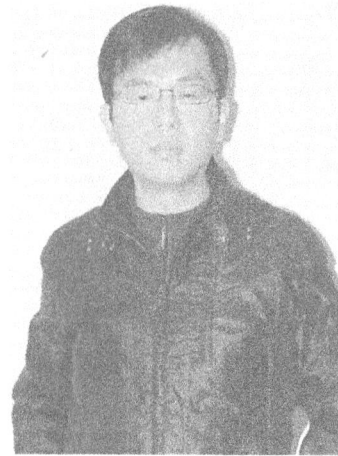
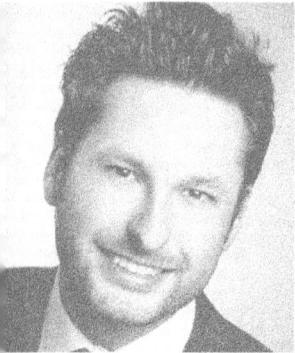
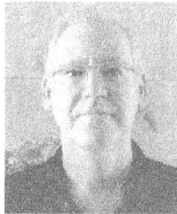

IntechOpen

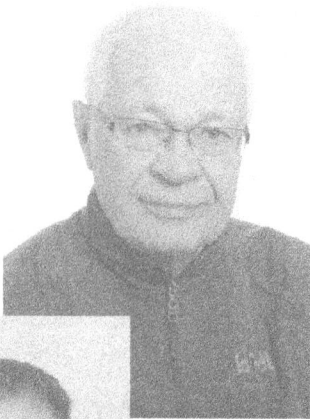
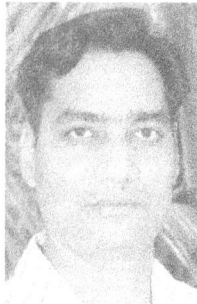
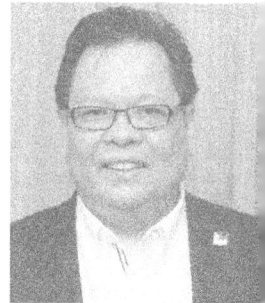
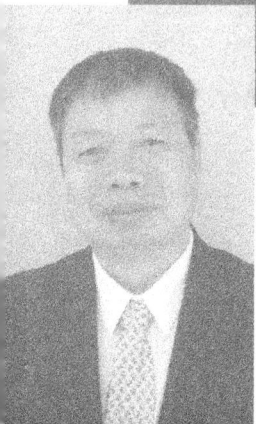
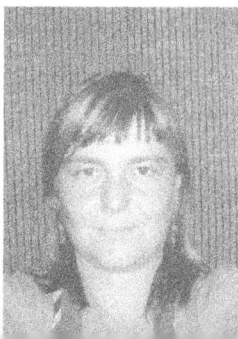
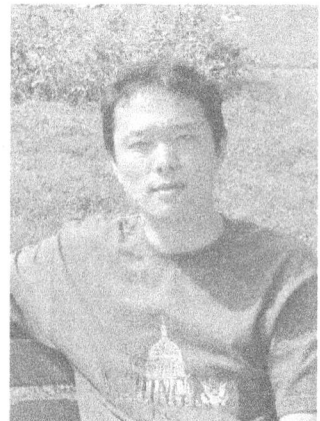

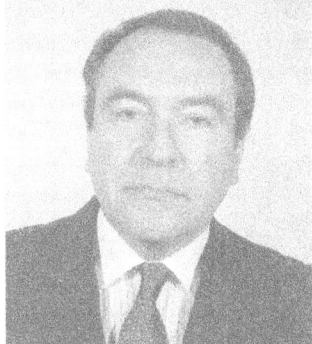

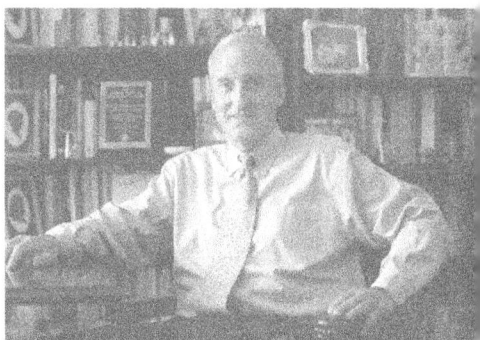

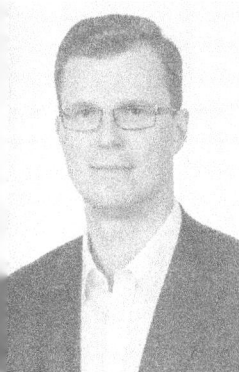

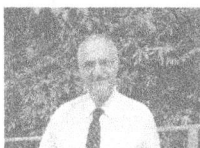

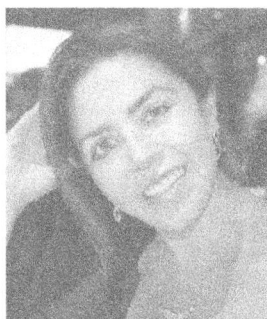

Supporting open minds since 2005

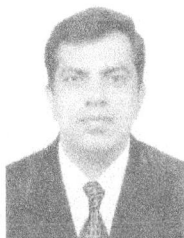

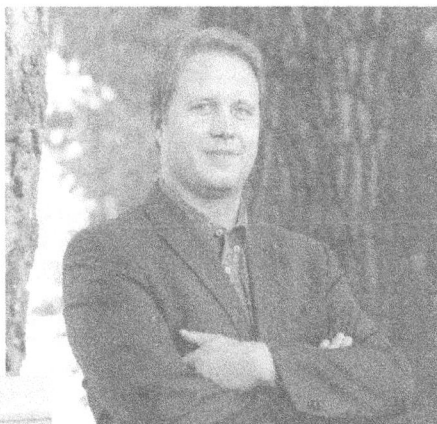

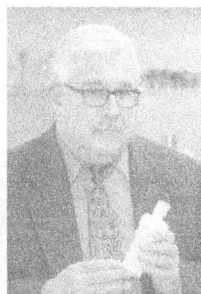

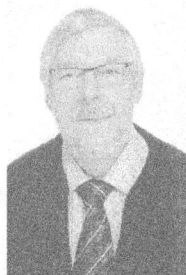

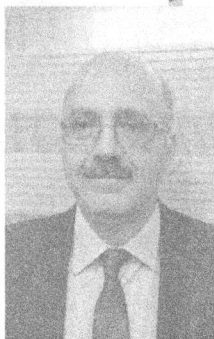

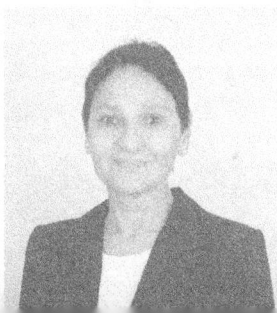

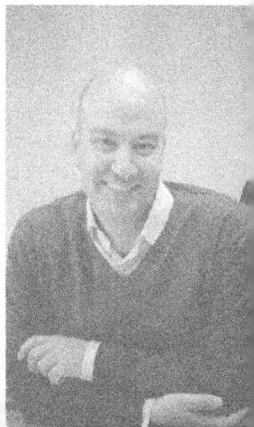

Pneumonia
http://dx.doi.org/10.5772/intechopen.73895
Edited by Nima Rezaei

Contributors
José de Jesús Olivares-Trejo, Maria Elizbeth Alvarez-Sánchez, Thang Nguyen, Kien T. Nguyen, Suol T. Pham, Thu P. M. Vo, Chu X. Duong, Dyah A. Perwitasari, Ngoc H. K. Truong, Dung T. H. Quach, Thao N. P. Nguyen, Van T. T. Duong, Phuong M. Nguyen, Thao H. Nguyen, Katja Taxis, Sachin M. Patil, Timothy R. Borgogna, Jovanka M. Voyich, Nima Rezaei, Aysan Moeinafshar

Notice
Statements and opinions expressed in the chapters are these of the individual contributors and not necessarily those of the editors or publisher. No responsibility is accepted for the accuracy of information contained in the published chapters. The publisher assumes no responsibility for any damage or injury to persons or property arising out of the use of any materials, instructions, methods or ideas contained in the book.

First published in London, United Kingdom, 2022 by IntechOpen
IntechOpen is the global imprint of INTECHOPEN LIMITED, registered in England and Wales, registration number: 11086078, 5 Princes Gate Court, London, SW7 2QJ, United Kingdom
Printed in Croatia

British Library Cataloguing-in-Publication Data
A catalogue record for this book is available from the British Library

Additional hard and PDF copies can be obtained from orders@intechopen.com

Pneumonia
Edited by Nima Rezaei
p. cm.

This title is part of the Infectious Diseases Book Series, Volume 13
Topic: Viral Infectious Diseases
Series Editor: Alfonso J. Rodriguez-Morales
Topic Editor: Shailendra K. Saxena

Print ISBN 978-1-83968-638-2
Online ISBN 978-1-83968-639-9
eBook (PDF) ISBN 978-1-83968-640-5
ISSN 2631-6188

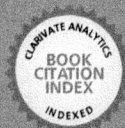

IntechOpen Book Series

Infectious Disease

Volume 13

Aims and Scope of the Series

This series will provide a comprehensive overview of recent research trends in various Infectious Diseases (as per the most recent Baltimore classification). Topics will include general overviews of infections, immunopathology, diagnosis, treatment, epidemiology, etiology, and current clinical recommendations for managing infectious diseases. Ongoing issues, recent advances, and future diagnostic approaches and therapeutic strategies will also be discussed. This book series will focus on various aspects and properties of infectious diseases whose deep understanding is essential for safeguarding the human race from losing resources and economies due to pathogens.

Meet the Series Editor

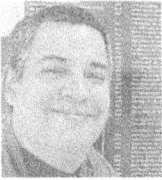

Dr. Rodriguez-Morales is an expert in tropical and emerging diseases, particularly zoonotic and vector-borne diseases (especially arboviral diseases). He is the president of the Travel Medicine Committee of the Pan-American Infectious Diseases Association (API), as well as the president of the Colombian Association of Infectious Diseases (ACIN). He is a member of the Committee on Tropical Medicine, Zoonoses, and Travel Medicine of ACIN. He is a vice-president of the Latin American Society for Travel Medicine (SLAMVI) and a Member of the Council of the International Society for Infectious Diseases (ISID). Since 2014, he has been recognized as a Senior Researcher, at the Ministry of Science of Colombia. He is a professor at the Faculty of Medicine of the Fundacion Universitaria Autonoma de las Americas, in Pereira, Risaralda, Colombia. He is an External Professor, Master in Research on Tropical Medicine and International Health, Universitat de Barcelona, Spain. He is also a professor at the Master in Clinical Epidemiology and Biostatistics, Universidad Científica del Sur, Lima, Peru. In 2021 he has been awarded the "Raul Isturiz Award" Medal of the API. Also, in 2021, he was awarded with the "Jose Felix Patiño" Asclepius Staff Medal of the Colombian Medical College, due to his scientific contributions to COVID-19 during the pandemic. He is currently the Editor in Chief of the journal Travel Medicine and Infectious Diseases. His Scopus H index is 47 (Google Scholar H index, 68).

Meet the Volume Editor

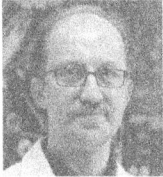

Professor Nima Rezaei obtained an MD from Tehran University of Medical Sciences, Iran. He also obtained an MSc in Molecular and Genetic Medicine, and a Ph.D. in Clinical Immunology and Human Genetics from the University of Sheffield, UK. He also completed a short-term fellowship in Pediatric Clinical Immunology and Bone Marrow Transplantation at Newcastle General Hospital, England. Dr. Rezaei is a Full Professor of Immunology and Vice Dean of International Affairs and Research, at the School of Medicine, Tehran University of Medical Sciences, and the co-founder and head of the Research Center for Immunodeficiencies. He is also the founding president of the Universal Scientific Education and Research Network (USERN). Dr. Rezaei has directed more than 100 research projects and has designed and participated in several international collaborative projects. He is an editor, editorial assistant, or editorial board member of more than forty international journals. He has edited more than 50 international books, presented more than 500 lectures/posters in congresses/meetings, and published more than 1,100 scientific papers in international journals.

Contents

Preface

Pneumonia is an infectious disease of the pulmonary alveoli caused by bacteria, viruses, and fungi. Pneumonia affects all age groups, although children and the elderly are more susceptible. Patterns of involvement of the lung tissue and the underlying pathogens vary widely among patients and can be divided into three groups: community-acquired pneumonia (CAP), hospital-acquired pneumonia (HAP), and ventilation-associated pneumonia (VAP). Of these, VAP and HAP are important causes of death, especially among hospitalized patients.

Pneumonia infections lead to extensive morbidity and mortality, particularly during this time of the COVID-19 pandemic, as the virus has been an important cause of complications in hospitalized patients. Though palliative care and antibiotic regimens have proven to positively affect management and survival in cases of pneumonia, a deeper understanding of the course and pathology of the disease, its underlying causes, and its mechanisms can vastly improve therapeutic approaches and patient survival.

This book contains five chapters, beginning with a brief introduction to pneumonia in Chapter 1. Chapter 2 discusses HAP, Chapter 3 addresses drug-related issues in pneumonia infections, Chapter 4 examines secondary bacterial infections in viral pneumonia, and Chapter 5 discusses issues such as iron acquisition in pneumococci.

We are indebted to the contributing authors for their excellent chapters and dedication to this project.

Nima Rezaei, MD, Ph.D.
Research Center for Immunodeficiencies,
Children's Medical Center,
Tehran University of Medical Sciences,
Tehran, Iran

Chapter 1

Introductory Chapter: Pneumonia

Aysan Moeinafshar and Nima Rezaei

1. Introduction

Pneumonia is an umbrella term regarding a variety of syndromes with different etiologies and refers to infection of the lung parenchyma. Pneumonia can be caused by a variety of microorganisms including bacterial, viral, and fungal pathogens [1]. Bacterial pneumonia can be divided into typical and atypical infections. Typical pneumonia is caused by microorganisms with the possibility of culturing on standard media or observation using gram staining techniques, such as *Streptococcus pneumonia*, *Staphylococcus aureus, Haemophylus influenza, Moraxella catarrhalis,* Group A streptococci, and gram-negative bacteria (both anaerobic and aerobic species). Atypical pneumonia is caused by pathogens that do not fit the aforementioned criteria; such as *Mycoplasma pneumoniae, Chlamydia pneumoniae,* and *Legionella* [2]. A variety of viruses, of both RNA and DNA virus families, can lead to pneumonia characteristics in patients. Some examples of these viruses include respiratory syncytial virus (RSV), rhinovirus, influenza viruses, parainfluenza viruses, adenovirus, varicella-zoster virus (VZV), cytomegalovirus (CMV), especially in HIV-infected patients, measles, and coronavirus family [3]. Fungal infections, though mostly overlooked, are important sources of pneumonia in immunocompromised patients. Some of the important organisms in this group include *Histoplasma, Blastomyces,* and *Coccidioides* [4].

2. Types of pneumonia

Pneumonia is classified into three groups based on etiology, disease characteristics, and clinical setting of the pathogen transmission. These subtypes include community-acquired pneumonia (CAP), hospital-acquired pneumonia (HAP), and ventilator-associated pneumonia (VAP) [1].

CAP is a type of pneumonia that is acquired in a community setting, caused by both atypical and typical bacterial organisms, viruses, and fungi [1, 5]. HAP is considered a type of pneumonia acquired 48 h after hospital admission, with no incubation at time of admission [6]. On the other hand, VAP is a pneumonia acquired in patients under endotracheal incubation 48 h after the procedure [7]. The underlying pathogens responsible for HAP and VAP include gram-negative bacilli (*Escherichia coli*, *Pseudomonas Aeruginosa, Acinetobacter, Enterobacter, Klebsiella,* etc.) and gram-positive cocci such as *S. aureus* [8]. Also, aspiration of both small (micro-aspiration) and large (macro-aspiration) amounts of oropharyngeal and upper gastrointestinal secretions is responsible for aspiration pneumonia, which accounts for approximately 5–15% of CAP cases [9].

Pneumonia's pattern of pulmonary involvement in these infectious diseases varies widely and can be categorized into lobar pneumonia, lobular pneumonia, and focal/diffused interstitial pneumonia [10].

Pneumonia subtype	CAP	HAP	Aspiration pneumonia
Risk factors	• Age < 5 • Age > 65 + comorbidities • Male gender • Immunocompromised • Life style (smoking, etc.) • Prematurity[p] • Household air pollution[p] • Ambient particulate matter[p] • Suboptimal breast feeding[p] • Pulmonary disease[A] • DM[A] • CVD[A] • Chronic liver disease[A]	• Male gender • Burns, trauma, surgery • History of antibiotic therapy • Malnutrition • Disease severity • Virulent pathogens in oropharynx • Pulmonary aspiration (and predisposing conditions to pulmonary aspiration) • ARDS	• Impaired swallowing • Decreased consciousness • Impaired cough reflex
References	[11]	[11]	[11]

Table 1.
Rrisk factors of pneumonia. (DM = diabetes mellitus, CVD = cardiovascular disease, ARDS = acute respiratory distress syndrome, p superscript: pediatric cases, A superscript: adult cases).

Risk factors predisposing patients to each of these pneumonia subtypes are summarized in **Table 1**.

3. Disease burden

The results of the Etiology of Pneumonia in the Community (EPIC) study in the united states indicated the annual incidence of CAP to be 2.4 cases per 1000 adults, mostly in age groups of >65 years old [12]. Similar studies in Europe estimated the annual incidence to be 1.07–1.2 cases per 1000 people [13]. The annual incidence of HAP is about 5–10 patients per 1000 hospital admissions worldwide and VAP cases include 10–25% of patients under ventilation [14].

Mortality of CAP in outpatient care, hospital wards, and ICU is <1%, 4–18%, and up to 50% respectively [15–17]. HAP and VAP are the most common causes of death in hospital-acquired infections with global mortality rates of 20–10% and 20–50% respectively [18–22].

4. Pathophysiology

Inability of the immune system in clearance of pathogens from the lower respiratory system is the basis for the incidence of pneumonia [23]. In addition to the pathogens, both local and systemic immune responses lead to parenchymal damage, constitutional symptoms, fluid congestion, pus formation in lungs, and reduction in alveolar compliance [24].

Pathological findings throughout this process consist of four stages including congestion, due to intra-alveolar edema, red hepatization, gray hepatization, both with characteristics of increased firmness of the parenchyma, and resolution [25].

5. Diagnosis

Most important symptoms stated by patients include fever, chills, diaphoresis, fatigue, myalgia, malaise, productive or non-productive coughs, dyspnea, and pleuritic chest pain [23]. Clinical data used in the definition of pneumonia include symptoms of acute lower respiratory tract disease for periods of less than 7 days, minimum of one systemic symptom, and newly appeared signs in chest examination unexplained by other conditions. Along with clinical criteria, laboratory tests, such as complete blood count (CBC), serum electrolytes, procalcitonin levels, renal and liver function tests, and radiologic findings, such as consolidations, abnormal silhouettes, opacities, and infiltrates, are also of importance in defining pneumonia [26].

6. Management

Management of CAP is carried out after a risk stratification process mostly using CURB-65 criteria. This scale consists of five criteria; Confusion, Uremia (BUN>20 mg/dl), respiratory rate > 30/minute, blood pressure < 90/60 mmHg, and ages>65 years. Treatments of HAP and VAP take more time and are more complicated. First-line treatment of pneumonia includes empirical antibiotic therapy using broad-spectrum antibiotics [1].

Figure 1 summarizes the approaches in the management of pneumonia.

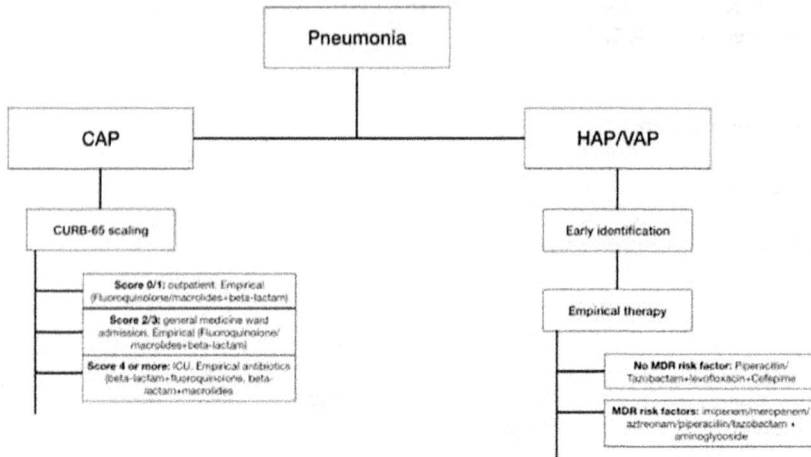

Figure 1.
Approach to pneumonia [1].

Author details

Aysan Moeinafshar[1,2,3] and Nima Rezaei[3,4,5]*

1 Cancer Immunology Project Interest Group (CIP), Universal Scientific Education and Research Network (USERN), Tehran, Iran

2 School of Medicine, Tehran University of Medical Sciences, Tehran, Iran

3 Network of Immunity in Infection, Malignancy and Autoimmunity (NIIMA), Universal Scientific Education and Research Network (USERN), Tehran, Iran

4 Research Center for Immunodeficiencies, Children's Medical Center, Tehran University of Medical Sciences, Tehran, Iran

5 Department of Immunology, School of Medicine, Tehran University of Medical Sciences, Tehran, Iran

*Address all correspondence to: rezaei_nima@yahoo.com

IntechOpen

References

[1] Jain V, Vashisht R, Yilmaz G, Bhardwaj A. Pneumonia Pathology. FL: Treasure Island; 2021

[2] Sattar SBA, Sharma S. Bacterial Pneumonia. FL: Treasure Island; 2021

[3] Freeman AM, Leigh Townes RJ. Viral Pneumonia. FL: Treasure Island; 2021

[4] Hage CA, Knox KS, Wheat LJ. Endemic mycoses: Overlooked causes of community acquired pneumonia. Respiratory Medicine. 2012;**106**(6): 769-776

[5] Mandell LA, Wunderink RG, Anzueto A, Bartlett JG, Campbell GD, Dean NC, et al. Infectious Diseases Society of America/American Thoracic Society consensus guidelines on the management of community-acquired pneumonia in adults. Clinical Infectious Diseases: An Offical Publication Infectious Diseases Soical American. 2007;**44**(Suppl 2):S27-S72

[6] Kalil AC, Metersky ML, Klompas M, Muscedere J, Sweeney DA, Palmer LB, et al. Executive summary: Management of adults with hospital-acquired and ventilator-associated pneumonia: 2016 clinical practice guidelines by the Infectious Diseases Society of America and the American Thoracic Society. Clinical Infectious Diseases: An Offical Publication Infectious Diseases Soical American. 2016;**63**(5):575-582

[7] Canadian Critical Care Trials Group. A randomized trial of diagnostic techniques for ventilator-associated pneumonia. The New England Journal of Medicine. Dec 2006;**355**(25):2619-2630

[8] Jones RN. Microbial etiologies of hospital-acquired bacterial pneumonia and ventilator-associated bacterial pneumonia. Clinical Infectious Diseases: An Offical Publication Infectious Diseases Soical American. 2010; **51**(Suppl 1):S81-S87

[9] Mandell LA, Niederman MS. Aspiration pneumonia. The New England Journal of Medicine. 2019;**380**(7):651-663

[10] Gharib AM, Stern EJ. Radiology of pneumonia. The Medical Clinics of North America. 2001;**85**(6):1461-1491

[11] Torres A, Cilloniz C, Niederman MS, Menéndez R, Chalmers JD, Wunderink RG, et al. Pneumonia. Nature Reviews Disease Primers [Internet]. 2021;**7**(1):25. DOI: 10.1038/s41572-021-00259-0

[12] Jain S, Self WH, Wunderink RG, Fakhran S, Balk R, Bramley AM, et al. Community-acquired pneumonia requiring hospitalization among US adults. The New England Journal of Medicine. 2015;**373**(5):415-427

[13] Torres A, Peetermans WE, Viegi G, Blasi F. Risk factors for community-acquired pneumonia in adults in Europe: A literature review. Thorax. 2013;**68**(11):1057-1065

[14] Torres A, Niederman MS, Chastre J, Ewig S, Fernandez-Vandellos P, Hanberger H, et al. International ERS/ESICM/ESCMID/ALAT guidelines for the management of hospital-acquired pneumonia and ventilator-associated pneumonia: Guidelines for the management of hospital-acquired pneumonia (HAP)/ventilator-associated pneumonia (VAP) of the European Respiratory Society (ERS), European Society of Intensive Care Medicine (ESICM), European Society of Clinical Microbiology and Infectious Diseases (ESCMID) and Asociación Latinoamericana del Tórax (ALAT). The European Respiratory Journal. 2017;**50**(3):1700582

[15] Arnold FW, Wiemken TL, Peyrani P, Ramirez JA, Brock GN. Mortality differences among hospitalized patients

with community-acquired pneumonia in three world regions: Results from the Community-Acquired Pneumonia Organization (CAPO) International Cohort Study. Respiratory Medicine. 2013;**107**(7):1101-1111

[16] Heo JY, Song JY. Disease burden and etiologic distribution of community-acquired pneumonia in adults: Evolving epidemiology in the era of pneumococcal conjugate vaccines. Infection & Chemotherapy. 2018; **50**(4):287-300

[17] Cillóniz C, Ewig S, Polverino E, Marcos MA, Prina E, Sellares J, et al. Community-acquired pneumonia in outpatients: Aetiology and outcomes. The European Respiratory Journal. 2012;**40**(4):931-938

[18] Magill SS, Edwards JR, Bamberg W, Beldavs ZG, Dumyati G, Kainer MA, et al. Multistate point-prevalence survey of health care–associated infections. The New England Journal of Medicine. 2014;**370**(13):1198-1208

[19] Micek ST, Chew B, Hampton N, Kollef MH. A case-control study assessing the impact of nonventilated hospital-acquired pneumonia on patient outcomes. Chest. 2016;**150**(5): 1008-1014

[20] Melsen WG, Rovers MM, Groenwold RHH, Bergmans DCJJ, Camus C, Bauer TT, et al. Attributable mortality of ventilator-associated pneumonia: A meta-analysis of individual patient data from randomised prevention studies. The Lancet Infectious Diseases. 2013;**13**(8):665-671

[21] Barbier F, Andremont A, Wolff M, Bouadma L. Hospital-acquired pneumonia and ventilator-associated pneumonia: Recent advances in epidemiology and management. Current Opinion in Pulmonary Medicine. 2013;**19**(3):216-228

[22] Bassetti M, Righi E, Vena A, Graziano E, Russo A, Peghin M. Risk stratification and treatment of ICU-acquired pneumonia caused by multidrug-resistant/extensively drug-resistant/pandrug-resistant bacteria. Current Opinion in Critical Care. 2018;**24**(5):385-393

[23] Kaysin A, Viera AJ. Community-acquired pneumonia in adults: Diagnosis and management. American Family Physician. 2016;**94**(9):698-706

[24] Cilloniz C, Martin-Loeches I, Garcia-Vidal C, San Jose A, Torres A. Microbial etiology of pneumonia: Epidemiology, diagnosis and resistance patterns. International Journal of Molecular Sciences. Dec 2016;**17**(12):2120

[25] Kradin RL, Digumarthy S. The pathology of pulmonary bacterial infection. Seminars in Diagnostic Pathology. 2017;**34**(6):498-509

[26] Ticona JH, Zaccone VM, McFarlane IM. Community-acquired pneumonia: A focused review. American Journal of Medical Case Reports. 2021;**9**(1):45-52. Available from: https://pubmed.ncbi.nlm.nih.gov/33313398 [Accessed: April 11, 2020]

Chapter 2

Hospital-Acquired Pneumonia

Sachin M. Patil

Abstract

Pneumonia acquired during hospitalization is called nosocomial pneumonia (NP). Nosocomial pneumonia is divided into two types. Hospital-acquired pneumonia (HAP) refers to hospital-acquired pneumonia, whereas ventilator-associated pneumonia (VAP) refers to ventilator-associated pneumonia. Most clinical literature stresses VAP's importance and associated mortality and morbidity, whereas HAP is not given enough attention even while being the most common cause of NP. HAP, like VAP, carries a high mortality and morbidity. HAP is the commonest cause of mortality from hospital-acquired infections. HAP is a common determinant for intensive care unit (ICU) admits with respiratory failure. Recent research has identified definite risk factors responsible for HAP. If these are prevented or modified, the HAP incidence can be significantly decreased with improved clinical outcomes and lesser utilization of the health care resources. The prevention approach will need multiple strategies to address the issues. Precise epidemiological data on HAP is deficient due to limitations of the commonly used diagnostic measures. The diagnostic modalities available in HAP are less invasive than VAP. Recent infectious disease society guidelines have stressed the importance of HAP by removing healthcare-associated pneumonia as a diagnosis. Specific differences exist between HAP and VAP, which are gleaned over in this chapter.

Keywords: hospital-acquired pneumonia (HAP), ventilator-associated pneumonia (VAP), ICU, prevention

1. Introduction

Nosocomial pneumonia (NP) that occurs during a patient's hospital course has been subclassified into hospital-acquired pneumonia (HAP) and ventilator-associated pneumonia (VAP). As per the latest Infectious Diseases Society of America (IDSA) and American Thoracic Society guidelines (ATS) [1], the category healthcare-associated pneumonia (HCAP) has been abandoned. The term NP and HAP should not be used interchangingly as before. HAP should be used only for pneumonia that occurs >48 h after admission to a hospital. VAP refers to pneumonia occurring >48 h post-intubation [2]. HAP is the most frequent hospital-acquired infection (HAI) [3]. As per the latest study done in the United States of America (USA), HAP prevalence in ICU was more frequent than VAP, and more than 75% of these patients developed severe respiratory failure due to pneumonia resulting in intubation and mechanical ventilatory support [4]. It is unknown whether the above trend is similar across all medical centers in the USA or is observed only in a few medical centers. Tertiary medical centers may have a different prevalence rate than other medical centers due to the higher presence of immunosuppressed patients (post-transplant). The lack of effective HAP surveillance systems in the

USA and other countries adds to this tenuous issue. Also, the lack of definitive diagnostic criteria makes it difficult to identify HAP patients on the floor and in intensive care units, as fever and cough can have multiple diagnostic possibilities postadmission to a hospital.

2. Epidemiology

HAP can occur in both patients with or without risk factors, and it is critical to realize that all acute care patients have an increased risk of HAP [5]. Specific patient subsets carry an increased risk than others, including elderly patients, chronic lung, cardiac and renal disease, hepatic cirrhosis, obesity, diabetes mellitus, cancer, neurological conditions such as stroke and dementia, malnutrition, and immunosuppressed patients [6, 7]. Specific therapeutic intervention modalities, including medications and procedures such as intubation, gastric tube placements, can increase the risk of HAP. Clinical literature on HAP inside the ICU is suboptimal, whereas on HAP outside the ICU is minuscule. NP accounts for around 21 admits per 1000 admissions to a hospital [8]. NP is responsible for close to 22% of HAI in the USA, and about 61% are HAP compared to VAP [9]. NP results in significant clinical outcomes such as increased healthcare costs, extended hospital stay, excess utilization of health care resources, and higher mortality and morbidity [10]. The actual prevalence rates of HAP and VAP are unknown; however, recent studies allude to a greater prevalence of HAP than VAP by a ratio of close to 2:1 in favor of HAP [11, 12]. A recent state study from Pennsylvania revealed that HAP risk factors and resulting complications are identical to those seen in VAP but were associated with an unfavorable higher economic cost and similar mortality [11]. Recent studies indicate an approximate incidence of 1.22 to 8.9 per 1000 patient days [5, 6, 9, 13, 14]. The total acute care cost for HAP is close to 40,000 dollars, with a hospital stay of 4 to 15.9 days, and the HAP influence on mortality was more significant than VAP [11, 13, 14]. Also, HAP patients, due to their increased occurrence, had a net increased economic cost than VAP and a higher need for postdischarge care [11, 14]. However, this cost did not include the interinstitutional transfer costs involved [14].

3. Etiology and risk factors

As patients diagnosed with HAP are not intubated, they face multiple challenges, including an inability to perform minimally invasive procedures to obtain microbiological specimens from the lower airway leading to the absence of microbiological data and ineffective initial antimicrobial treatment. In a large European trial involving 27 ICU units among HAP patients, only 54.8% of patients had positive microbiology data. *Enterobacteriaceae* are the most frequent cause, followed by *Staphylococcus aureus*, *Pseudomonas aeruginosa*, and *Acinetobacter baumannii* [15]. In another study, the microbial causes were similar between HAP and VAP except for an increased occurrence of *Streptococcus pneumoniae* in HAP patients [16]. 80% of cases were caused by *Klebsiella spp.*, *Enterobacter spp.*, *Escherichia coli*, *Staphylococcus aureus*, *Acinetobacter spp.*, and *Pseudomonas aeruginosa* per the clinical data registered in the antimicrobial surveillance program SENTRY [17]. Also, in this study, severe sepsis and pneumonia occurred only in centers with >25% Multi-drug Resistance (MDR) prevalence, even in those lacking risk elements and early pneumonia. Upon reviewing the data mentioned above, gram-negative bacilli (GNB) cause most of these infections and are frequently resistant to antibiotics, making an empirical antibiotic decision difficult. In transplant patients, the microbial etiology differs based on the transplant type, duration post-transplant, and the antirejection mediations they are currently on. In hematopoietic stem cell transplants, bacterial causes were the highest, followed by fungal and viral [18]. Among the bacterial causes, the most common cause was *Escherichia coli*, *Pseudomonas aeruginosa*, and *Streptococcus pneumoniae*. GNB was the most frequent in solid organ transplants, especially *Pseudomonas aeruginosa*, *Enterobacteriaceae*, followed by *Staphylococcus aureus*, often with an MDR profile [19]. The microorganisms responsible vary based on the patient population, MDR risk factors, geographical location, and duration of hospital stay before disease onset [2]. An essential factor to recognize is identifying any Multi-drug resistance organism (MDRO) risk factors, clinical severity, and local ecology before empirical antibiotic therapy. **Tables 1–3** reveals the risk factors for

Invasive MSSA[*] infection risk factors	MRSA[**] HAP risk factors
1. Cardiac disease	1. Tobacco abuse
2. Diabetes mellitus	2. Illicit drug abuse
3. Cancer	3. Recent hospitalization <90 days
4. Chronic obstructive pulmonary disease	4. Recent antibiotics
5. Hemodialysis	5. Chronic obstructive pulmonary disease
6. Stroke	6. Liver disease
7. Intravenous drug abuse	7. HIV infection
8. Rheumatoid arthritis	
9. Human immunodeficiency viral infection	
10. Peritoneal dialysis	
11. Solid organ transplantation	
12. Systemic lupus erythematosus	

"Created with BioRender."
[*]*MSSA—Methicillin-sensitive* Staphylococcus aureus.
[**]*MRSA—Methicillin-resistant* Staphylococcus aureus.

Table 1.
Invasive MSSA infection risk factors, MRSA HAP risk factors.

1. Prior infection with *pseudomonas spp.*
2. *Pseudomonas spp.* colonization
3. Very severe COPD
4. Bronchiectasis
5. Tracheostomy
6. Neutropenia
7. Burns
8. Cystic fibrosis
9. Long term acute care residents

"Created with BioRender."

Table 2.
Pseudomonas spp. *HAP risk factors.*

1. Long term acute care residents
2. Prior colonization/infection
3. Longer hospital duration stay
4. Prior antibiotics use
5. Acinetobacter skin infections
6. Poor healthcare worker hygeine
7. Contamined procedure equipment

"Created with BioRender."

Table 3.
Acinetobacter spp. *HAP risk factors.*

Staphylococcus aureus [20, 21], *Pseudomonas aeruginosa* [22], and *Acinetobacter baumannii* [23–26].

A prospective study has revealed the intrinsic and extrinsic risk factors for HAP in non-ICU patients, as shown in **Table 4** [6]. Demographically age > 60 years and males are at higher risk of acquiring HAP.

4. Pathophysiology

The upper airway and the oropharynx are usually colonized with nonpathogenic microorganisms, including the virulent *Staphylococcus aureus* and *Streptococcus pneumoniae*, and anaerobes. The lower airway microbiome is not entirely void of bacteria, as thought before [27]. The lower airway microbiome changes during

Intrinsic risk factors	Extrinsic risk factors
1. Cancer	1. Duration of hospitalization >5 days
2. Chronic obstructive pulmonary disease	2. Prior antibiotic therapy
3. Diabetes mellitus	3. H2 antagonist
4. Congestive heart failure	4. Steroids
5. Chronic renal failure	5. Antacids
6. Depression	6. Chemotherapy
7. Neutropenia	7. Prior endotracheal intubation
8. Obesity	8. Nasogstric tube
9. Malnutrition	9. Nebulization
10. Liver cirrhosis	10. Abdominal surgery
11. Human immunodeficiency virus infection	11. Prior ICU admission
	12. Thoracic surgery
	13. Head and neck surgery
	14. Tracheotomy

"Created with BioRender.com."

Table 4.
Intrinsic and extrinsic risk factors for HAP in non ICU patients.

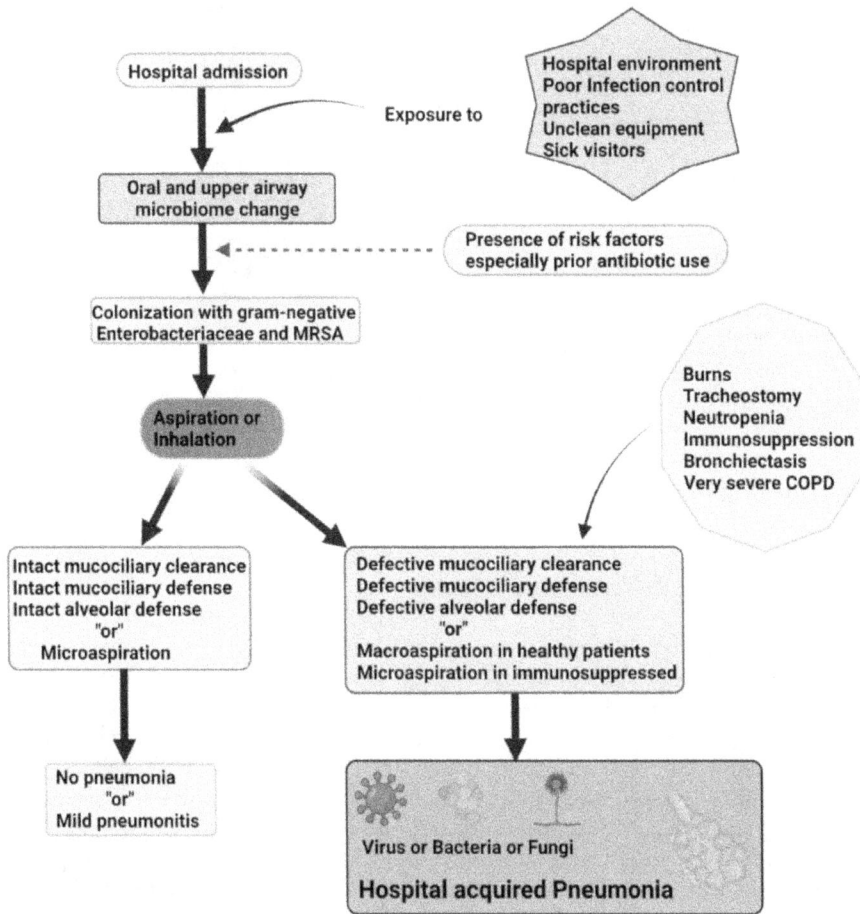

Figure 1.
Pathophysiology of HAP.

chronic lung disease or prolonged immunosuppression. Within a few days post-admission, the upper airway and the oropharynx flora changes on exposure to the hospital ecology and get colonized with MRSA (*Methicillin-sensitive Staphylococcus aureus*) and GNB [28, 29]. Most HAP occurs after aspiration of the oropharyngeal flora except for few bacterial microorganisms, viral and fungal microorganisms, which occur via respiratory droplets or inhalation. Once inhaled or aspirated, the intact mucociliary clearance, mucociliary and alveolar defense will try to clear it up [30–33]. They are often successful, but in cases with a large aspiration in a healthy patient or microaspiration in an immunosuppressed individual, the protective mechanisms are overwhelmed and result in HAP with significant inflammation and systemic signs. This entire process has been outlined in **Figure 1**.

5. Clinical features

The clinical features of HAP have been summarized as follows in **Table 5**.

Clinical symptoms	Clinical signs
1. Fever	1. Tachycardia
2. Dyspnea	2. Hypotension
3. Cough	3. Tachypnea
4. Tachypnea	4. Hypoxia
5. Chest pain	5. Rales
6. Purulent sputum	6. Wheezing
7. Hypothermia	7. Use of accessory respiratory muscles
8. Generalized weakness	8. Absent/decreased breath sounds
9. Confusion	9. Altered mental status

"Created with BioRender."

Table 5.
Clinical features of hospital-acquired pneumonia.

6. Diagnosis and differential diagnosis

Due to the lack of diagnostic criteria, clinical features need to be supplemented by imaging or laboratory tests for a HAP diagnosis. Imaging is often a portable or a two-view chest radiograph that reveals new pulmonary infiltrates, cavitation, abscess, or pleural effusion. Chest computed tomography (CT) is a gold standard in comparison and has better sensitivity than chest X-rays [34]. Recently, bedside ultrasound has been used to identify new pulmonary infiltrates with 94% sensitivity and 96% specificity [35]. A retrospective trial has revealed that biomarkers procalcitonin and C-reactive protein correlate well with HAP severity and could be a better prognostic marker for mortality and morbidity than neutrophil/lymphocyte count ratio [36]. A complete blood count may demonstrate leukocytosis. The differential count is essential in identifying any neutrophilia, neutropenia, eosinophilia, and a peripheral smear may demonstrate Dohle bodies that are more suggestive of ongoing infection. Microbiological workup can be invasive or noninvasive. Blood cultures with the help of MALDI BioTyper and FilmArray BCID can help rapidly identify the bacteria [37]. In transplant patients, a fungal blood culture would be ideal. Urine legionella and Streptococcal antigens can help identify the cause of pneumonia. Serum Aspergillus antigen assay and β-D-glucan assay is a must in transplant and immunosuppressed individuals when suspected. Nasopharyngeal swab polymerase chain reaction (PCR), also called a respiratory pathogen panel, can be utilized to identify some of the common respiratory bacterial and viral pathogens causing community-acquired pneumonia, which can also cause HAP due to significant exposure prior to admission and in the hospital.

The sputum gram stain, sputum specimen PCR, and culture should be done to identify the suspected etiological agent. If there is a lack of sputum, production then it can be induced by inhaled hypertonic saline. Sputum PCR using BioFire FilmArray Pneumonia or Pneumonia plus panel yields excellent sensitivity and specificity but must be adopted judiciously, and it could provide appropriate clinical information for antimicrobial stewardship [38, 39]. It can also detect atypical bacteria, common viral causes of pneumonia, common mechanisms of resistance and provide semiquantitative results for the common colonizers [40]. It provides valuable data for the clinician to deescalate the antibiotics to a narrow spectrum. This PCR test does not detect oral anaerobes, and they need to be considered with positive imaging and a negative PCR test to cover them with appropriate antibiotics. The PCR test should be done early in the clinical course to avoid false negatives and must be corroborated with the culture as much as possible. A sputum fungal culture or stain also might be helpful in transplant patients.

The invasive strategy involves performing a fibreoptic bronchoscopy, obtaining a bronchioalveolar lavage (BAL) sample, and performing BAL tests, including gram stain, fungal stain, cytology with methenamine stain, and quantitative culture (bacterial and fungal). BAL Aspergillus antigen assay, β-D-glucan assay, fungal and viral PCR assays can detect the causative agent in immunosuppressed or transplant patients. Invasive tests are done seldomly in stable patients as most of these patients are sick, unstable and the procedure may clinically deteriorate them [41]. If the patient during his clinical course gets intubated, then a BAL should be obtained to obtain more clinical information.

The betaLACTA test (BLT) detects GNB insensitivity to third-generation cephalosporins due to carbapenemases, ESBL (extended-spectrum beta-lactamases), and beta-lactamases from acquired AmpC carbapenemases in less than 20 min after exposure to respiratory bacterial cell pellets via chromogenic analysis [42]. The test detects GNB resistance via a colorimetric indicator and can quickly be used for antibiotic de-escalation [43]. It is currently being evaluated for its clinical efficaciousness in France's multicenter randomized controlled trial (RCT) called BLUE-CarbA [44].

A clinical diagnosis of HAP is currently considered with a new lung infiltrate and two of the four findings, including new-onset temperature > 38 degrees celsius, purulent sputum, and leukocytosis or leukopenia [45]. Most clinical diagnostic scores, including modified clinical pulmonary infection score (CPIS), the older National safety health network (NHSN) pneumonia definition, and the new infection-related Ventilator-associated complication (IVAC), have been used extensively in VAP and not in HAP. NHSN does suggest using the pneumonia definition for nonventilated adult patients for surveillance purposes (**Table 6**).

1. Two or more serial chest imaging test results with at least one of the following new and persistent or Progressive and persistent (Radiological criteria)
*Infiltrate/Consolidation/Cavitation
PLUS
2. Atleast one of the following (Systemic criteria)
• Fever (>38.0°C or > 100.4°F)
• Leukopenia (≤4000 WBC/mm^3) or leukocytosis (≥12,000 WBC/mm^3)
• For adults ≥70 years old, altered mental status with no other recognized cause
PLUS
3. And at least two of the following (Pulmonary criteria)
• New onset of purulent sputum or change in character of sputum, or increased respiratory secretions, or increased suctioning requirements
• New onset or worsening cough, or dyspnea, or tachypnea
• Rales6 or bronchial breath sounds
• Worsening gas exchange (for example: O$_2$ desaturations (for example: PaO$_2$/FiO$_2$ ≤ 240)7, increased oxygen requirements, or increased ventilator demand)

Table 6.
National health safety network definition of pneumonia (NHSN PNEU).

1. Pulmonary contusion
2. Pulmonary inhalation injuries
3. Atelectasis
4. Pleural effusion
5. Pulmonary edema
6. Pulmonary hemorrhage
7. Drug-induced pneumonitis
8. Pulomary infarct/embolism
9. Vasculitis
10. Primary or secondary pulmonary neoplasm

Table 7.
Differential diagnosis of HAP.

However, the long-term clinical utility of its use is unknown due to its lack of accuracy and consistency in VAP [46].

Clinical conditions that may simulate HAP and may need to be considered part of the differential diagnosis are mentioned in **Table** 7.

7. Treatment

Initial inappropriate antibiotic regimens and MDRO are independent indicators of ICU mortality and related to a longer mechanical ventilation duration [47]. Physicians always face a clinical scenario where they have to treat a patient with no lower respiratory specimen with the possibility of pending acute respiratory failure requiring mechanical ventilation [41]. Empirical antibiotic therapy can be based either on institutional epidemiology or a surveillance culture report updated annually. Although they yield similar results, the use of surveillance culture report results in reduced broad-spectrum antibiotics uses even in the presence of higher MDRO risk factors [48]. Individual patient risk factors need to be considered before an initial empirical regimen is started for HAP [49]. A suggestion is to use the local antibiogram in deciding the initial regimen. Most regimens include a broad-spectrum gram-positive coverage (vancomycin or linezolid) and a gram-negative coverage (carbapenem or fourth-generation cephalosporin or a piperacillin-tazobactam). It is prudent to use an antipseudomonal agent to cover gram-negative bacteria in the empirical regimen. MRSA screening of nares has a 96.1% negative predictive value for respiratory cultures [50]. Gram-positive bacterial coverage can be deescalated to MSSA coverage with a negative MRSA nasal screen if the clinical condition warrants it.

For de-escalation, at 48 to 72 h postadmission, procalcitonin plus C-reactive protein and a positive microbiological workup assist the clinical criteria [2]. De-escalation involves a transition from broad-spectrum to narrow-spectrum antimicrobial therapy. For atypical organism coverage, if suspected, rarely responsible for HAP, azithromycin or fluoroquinolone, or doxycycline can be used in addition to the empirical therapy. For *P. aeruginosa* HAP with no susceptibility results or absence of septic shock or high death risk, dual antipseudomonal coverage is indicated [2]. If the susceptibility pattern has resulted and in the absence of septic shock and increased risk of death, monotherapy is appropriate. *P. aeruginosa* HAP with carbapenemase resistance (CRE) can still be treated with ceftolozane/tazobactam combination as its primary resistance is via porin channels [51]. With ESBL GNB causing HAP, the recommended therapy is carbapenems with suggested alternatives, including ceftolozane/tazobactam combination. With *Acinetobacter spp.*, the treatment is based on antimicrobial susceptibility and usually involves more than one drug. CRE GNB is treated with Ceftazidime/avibactam, and Aztreonam is added to combination in GNB carrying Metallo-carbapenemase. The usual duration of treatment is around 7 days as in VAP with some exceptions, which include MSSA, MRSA, nonfermenting GNB such as *Pseudomonas, Stenotrophomonas, Acinetobacter*, and *Burkholderia spp.*, which have a higher rate of recurrence with 7 days of therapy (this data extrapolated from VAP studies) [52]. Regarding MSSA and MRSA HAP, the duration mentioned above is a recommended expert opinion due to the lack of RCTs on the course of therapy (7 vs. 14 days) [53]. Other exceptions to the seven-day course could be patients with immunosuppression and necrotizing pneumonia. Antimicrobial treatment should be based on the pharmacokinetics and pharmacodynamic data of the individual antimicrobial to avoid unwanted side effects.

8. Prevention

The utilization of any preventive measures to halt HAP should effectively alter the pathophysiology of the disease. Multiple measures have been carried out over the last few decades to prevent HAP or, preferably, VAP with variable degrees of success (**Table 8**).

Active measures taken	Effectiveness of measure
A. Exposure reduction: All the below-mentioned measures need further evaluation in HAP patients [54].	
Limit admission to hospital as much as possible	Increased hospitalization duration is associated with increased sepsis warning scores and increased exposure to HAP pathogens [55]. The risk in elderly patients increases at a rate of 0.3% per day [56]. Decreased duration of hospitalization results in decreased exposure and risk; however, this needs prospective assessment.
Healthcare worker and equipment hygiene	It prevents microbial spread between patients, health care workers, and essential equipment and improves VAP and catheter-associated bloodstream infection rates [57]. Stethoscopes and portable procedure equipment cleaning with chlorhexidine or alcohol-based sanitizer are ideal [58, 59]. The use of a portable stethoscope separately for each patient is another option [60]. Minimally invasive procedure equipment such as endoscopes and bronchoscopes should be sterilized with stringent protocols. Low compliance is frequent in healthcare workers and needs to be improved with structured educational programs and timely reinforcements [61].
Isolation measures	Standard isolation precautions such as universal gowns and gloves are ineffective in preventing the transmission of infections caused by MDRO [62]. However, they are highly effective in preventing *Clostridium difficile (C. difficile)* transmission [63]. Droplet precautions in hospitalized influenza infections prevent its spread.
B. Aspiration reduction: As mentioned above, the below-mentioned measures need validation in HAP patients.	
Prevent and reduce xerostomia	Xerostomia or oral dryness correlates with fever in dysphagia patients, but its association with HAP is unknown [64]. Also, the effect of xerostomia prevention and treatment with sialogogues on HAP incidence and prevalence is unknown [65].

Active measures taken	Effectiveness of measure
Timely identification of dysphagia	Identifying patients with a higher risk of dysphagia promptly by a higher screening adherence results in lower HAP rates [66]. This is especially important in patients with neurological disorders. Dysphagia evaluation by a speech therapist can lead to modified diets in specific population subsets with a lower incidence of pneumonia [67].
Feeding via enteral tubes	Jejunostomy tubes compared to gastric ones result in lower VAP and HAP rates [68]. The use of a motility agent has lead to variable results in a systematic review, and its benefit is questionable [69].
Patient position modification	A semi-recumbent position (30° to 45°) during feeding decreases acid reflux and the risk of aspiration with a decline in VAP rates [70].
Mobilization	Earlier mobilization stops the functional decline, improves airway clearance, and prevents HAP [71]. Family member's training helps in extending this benefit outside of the healthcare environment [72].
C. Active interventions	
Oral hygiene	Bad oral hygiene results in increased colonization with airway pathogens and periodontal disease [73]. It can diminish cough reflex and impair airway hygiene leading to pneumonia [74, 75]. Interventions to improve oral hygiene are the best known cost-effective preventive strategy for HAP [5, 76]. Adequate training of nursing staff in oral care practices is critical with timely reinforcements.
Decontamination of oral, digestive, and skin	Skin decontamination with chlorhexidine decreases VAP, HAI but its effect on HAP is unknown [77]. Oral decontamination with chlorhexidine diminishes VAP rates and increases mortality; however, its implication on HAP is unknown [12, 78]. Selective digestive decontamination (SDD) with oral, topical, and intravenous antibiotics decreased VAP and is thought to be adequate in HAP [79]. SDD use was in countries with lower antibiotic resistance levels, and its long-term effects are unknown [12].
Vaccination	Vaccination against hospital pathogens is ineffective [80], whereas monoclonal antibodies have shown promise adjunctively with antibiotics in early trials for *Staphylococcus aureus* and *Pseudomonas aeruginosa* [81].
Medications and other factors	As medications preventing gastric-acid secretions are linked to increased HAP rates, preventing their indiscriminate use is necessary [82]. Adequate glucose control preventing hypo and hyperglycemia is critical in halting airway colonization and pneumonia risk [83, 84]. Probiotics may decrease the HAP rate; however, they have not been evaluated in HAP.
Airway hygiene	When done preemptively in postoperative and hospitalized pneumonia patients, chest physical therapy has revealed modest preventive effects [85, 86].
Respiratory support	Noninvasive ventilation (NIV) decreased nosocomial pneumonia and improved outcomes in specific patient subsets [87]. Although it allows for better airway clearance and comfort, high-flow nasal cannula use did not decrease HAP incidence in two small randomized controlled trials [88, 89]. Recent helmet use in NIV did not decrease HAP rates compared to facemask [90].
Staffing practices	Increased nursing staff to patient ratio results in lower HAP and HAI rates [91]. The presence of daytime intensivists correlates with improved mortality overall [92]. The effect of 24 h physician staffing on the HAP rates is unknown.

Table 8.
HAP preventive measures.

A constant surveillance system absence regarding HAP has prevented effective detection and monitoring of HAP rates in the USA. An objective assessment is hampered by the lack of standard diagnostic criteria, microbiologic and diagnostic coding data [54]. Also, only a few preventive measures have been validated, and the remaining lack adequate clinical data for physicians to implement them successfully. It requires multidisciplinary team involvement for the effective implementation of these preventive measures.

9. Conclusion

The administratively coded data (ACD) used for billing is limited, and its accuracy is imprecise in HAP detection and surveillance [14]. A better approach to this problem will be to use proven assessed techniques, and this practice should be utilized in HAP detection. The approach should start with creating a specific diagnostic criterion followed by evidence-based guidelines to help in decreasing its incidence and prevalence with additional stress on earlier detection and prevention.

Acknowledgements

"No external funds were utilized in the manuscript preparation."

Conflict of interest

"The author declares no conflict of interest."

Notes/Thanks/Other declarations

"I thank the editor for letting me author this manuscript."

Acronyms and abbreviations

NP	Nosocomial pneumonia
HAP	Hospital-acquired pneumonia
VAP	Ventilator-associated pneumonia
ICU	Intensive care unit
IDSA	Infectious Diseases Society of America
HCAP	Healthcare-associated pneumonia
HAI	Hospital-acquired infections
USA	United States of America
MDR	Multi-drug Resistance
MDRO	Multi-drug Resistance Organism
HIV	Human Immunodeficiency virus
MSSA	Methicillin-sensitive *Staphylococcus aureus*
MRSA	Methicillin-resistant *Staphylococcus aureus*
COPD	Chronic obstructive pulmonary disease
GNB	Gram-negative bacilli
CT	Computed tomography

MALDI	Matrix-assisted laser desorption ionization
BCID	Blood Culture ID Panel
PCR	Polymerase chain reaction
BAL	Bronchioalveolar lavage
BLT	betaLACTA test
ESBL	Extended-spectrum beta-lactamase
RCT	Randomized controlled trial
CPIS	Clinical pulmonary infection score
NHSN	National health safety network
IVAC	Infection-related Ventilator-associated complication
CRE	Carbapenemase resistance
SDD	Selective digestive decontamination
NIV	Noninvasive ventilation
ACD	Administratively coded data

Author details

Sachin M. Patil
Infectious Disease Critical Care, University of Missouri, Columbia, MO, USA

*Address all correspondence to: drssmp1@gmail.com

IntechOpen

References

[1] Metlay JP, Waterer GW, Long AC, Anzueto A, Brozek J, Crothers K, et al. Diagnosis and treatment of adults with community-acquired pneumonia. An official clinical practice guideline of the american thoracic society and infectious diseases society of America. American Journal of Respiratory and Critical Care Medicine. 2019;**200**(7):e45-e67

[2] Kalil AC, Metersky ML, Klompas M, Muscedere J, Sweeney DA, Palmer LB, et al. Management of adults with hospital-acquired and ventilator-associated pneumonia: 2016 clinical practice guidelines by the infectious diseases society of America and the American thoracic society. Clinical Infectious Diseases. 2016;**63**(5):e61-e111

[3] Vincent JL, Rello J, Marshall J, Silva E, Anzueto A, Martin CD, et al. International study of the prevalence and outcomes of infection in intensive care units. Journal of the American Medical Association. 2009;**302**(21): 2323-2329

[4] Kett DH, Cano E, Quartin AA, Mangino JE, Zervos MJ, Peyrani P, et al. Implementation of guidelines for management of possible multidrug-resistant pneumonia in intensive care: An observational, multicentre cohort study. The Lancet Infectious Diseases. 2011;**11**(3):181-189

[5] Quinn B, Baker DL, Cohen S, Stewart JL, Lima CA, Parise C. Basic nursing care to prevent nonventilator hospital-acquired pneumonia. Journal of Nursing Scholarship. 2014;**46**(1):11-19

[6] Sopena N, Sabria M, Neunos SG. Multicenter study of hospital-acquired pneumonia in non-ICU patients. Chest. 2005;**127**(1):213-219

[7] Cilloniz C, Polverino E, Ewig S, Aliberti S, Gabarrus A, Menendez R, et al. Impact of age and comorbidity on cause and outcome in community-acquired pneumonia. Chest. 2013; **144**(3):999-1007

[8] Chawla R. Epidemiology, etiology, and diagnosis of hospital-acquired pneumonia and ventilator-associated pneumonia in Asian countries. American Journal of Infection Control. 2008;**36**(4 Suppl):S93-S100

[9] Magill SS, Edwards JR, Bamberg W, Beldavs ZG, Dumyati G, Kainer MA, et al. Multistate point-prevalence survey of health care-associated infections. The New England Journal of Medicine. 2014; **370**(13):1198-1208

[10] Eber MR, Laxminarayan R, Perencevich EN, Malani A. Clinical and economic outcomes attributable to health care-associated sepsis and pneumonia. Archives of Internal Medicine. 2010;**170**(4):347-353

[11] Davis J, Finley AE, editors. The breadth of hospital-acquired pneumonia: Nonventilated versus ventilated patients in Pennsylvania. Pennsylvania Patient Safety Advisory. 2012;**9**(3):99-105. Available from: http://patientsafety.pa.gov/ ADVISORIES/Documents/201209_99. pdf

[12] Torres A, Niederman MS, Chastre J, Ewig S, Fernandez-Vandellos P, Hanberger H, et al. International ERS/ ESICM/ESCMID/ALAT guidelines for the management of hospital-acquired pneumonia and ventilator-associated pneumonia: Guidelines for the management of hospital-acquired pneumonia (HAP)/ventilator-associated pneumonia (VAP) of the European Respiratory Society (ERS), European Society of Intensive Care Medicine (ESICM), European Society of Clinical Microbiology and Infectious Diseases (ESCMID) and Asociacion

Latinoamericana del Torax (ALAT). European Respiratory Journal. 2017; **50**(3):2

[13] Micek ST, Chew B, Hampton N, Kollef MH. A case-control study assessing the impact of nonventilated hospital-acquired pneumonia on patient outcomes. Chest. 2016;**150**(5): 1008-1014

[14] Giuliano KK, Baker D, Quinn B. The epidemiology of nonventilator hospital-acquired pneumonia in the United States. American Journal of Infection Control. 2018;**46**(3):322-327

[15] Koulenti D, Tsigou E, Rello J. Nosocomial pneumonia in 27 ICUs in Europe: Perspectives from the EU-VAP/CAP study. European Journal of Clinical Microbiology & Infectious Diseases. 2017;**36**(11):1999-2006

[16] Esperatti M, Ferrer M, Theessen A, Liapikou A, Valencia M, Saucedo LM, et al. Nosocomial pneumonia in the intensive care unit acquired by mechanically ventilated versus nonventilated patients. American Journal of Respiratory and Critical Care Medicine. 2010;**182**(12):1533-1539

[17] Jones RN. Microbial etiologies of hospital-acquired bacterial pneumonia and ventilator-associated bacterial pneumonia. Clinical Infectious Diseases. 2010;**51**(Suppl 1):S81-S87

[18] Aguilar-Guisado M, Jimenez-Jambrina M, Espigado I, Rovira M, Martino R, Oriol A, et al. Pneumonia in allogeneic stem cell transplantation recipients: A multicenter prospective study. Clinical Transplantation. 2011; **25**(6):E629-E638

[19] Giannella M, Munoz P, Alarcon JM, Mularoni A, Grossi P, Bouza E, et al. Pneumonia in solid organ transplant recipients: A prospective multicenter study. Transplant Infectious Disease. 2014;**16**(2):232-241

[20] Laupland KB, Church DL, Mucenski M, Sutherland LR, Davies HD. Population-based study of the epidemiology of and the risk factors for invasive Staphylococcus aureus infections. The Journal of Infectious Diseases. 2003;**187**(9):1452-1459

[21] Wooten DA, Winston LG. Risk factors for methicillin-resistant Staphylococcus aureus in patients with community-onset and hospital-onset pneumonia. Respiratory Medicine. 2013; **107**(8):1266-1270

[22] Restrepo MI, Babu BL, Reyes LF, Chalmers JD, Soni NJ, Sibila O, et al. Burden and risk factors for *Pseudomonas aeruginosa* community-acquired pneumonia: A multinational point prevalence study of hospitalised patients. European Respiratory Journal. 2018;**52**(2):2, 9, 10

[23] Turton JF, Shah J, Ozongwu C, Pike R. Incidence of acinetobacter species other than *A. baumannii* among clinical isolates of acinetobacter: Evidence for emerging species. Journal of Clinical Microbiology. 2010;**48**(4):1445-1449

[24] Thom KA, Johnson JK, Lee MS, Harris AD. Environmental contamination because of multidrug-resistant *Acinetobacter baumannii* surrounding colonized or infected patients. American Journal of Infection Control. 2011;**39**(9):711-715

[25] Wong D, Nielsen TB, Bonomo RA, Pantapalangkoor P, Luna B, Spellberg B. Clinical and pathophysiological overview of acinetobacter infections: A century of challenges. Clinical Microbiology Reviews. 2017;**30**(1):409-447

[26] Falagas ME, Rafailidis PI. Attributable mortality of *acinetobacter baumannii*: No longer a controversial issue. Critical Care. 2007;**11**(3):134

[27] Charlson ES, Bittinger K, Haas AR, Fitzgerald AS, Frank I, Yadav A, et al.

Topographical continuity of bacterial populations in the healthy human respiratory tract. American Journal of Respiratory and Critical Care Medicine. 2011;**184**(8):957-963

[28] Johanson WG Jr, Pierce AK, Sanford JP, Thomas GD. Nosocomial respiratory infections with gram-negative bacilli. The significance of colonization of the respiratory tract. Annals of Internal Medicine. 1972;**77**(5): 701-706

[29] Johanson WG, Pierce AK, Sanford JP. Changing pharyngeal bacterial flora of hospitalized patients. Emergence of gram-negative *bacilli*. The New England Journal of Medicine. 1969; **281**(21):1137-1140

[30] Ware SM, Aygun MG, Hildebrandt F. Spectrum of clinical diseases caused by disorders of primary cilia. Proceedings of the American Thoracic Society. 2011;**8**(5):444-450

[31] Voynow JA, Rubin BK. Mucins, mucus, and sputum. Chest. 2009;**135**(2): 505-512

[32] Parker D, Prince A. Innate immunity in the respiratory epithelium. American Journal of Respiratory Cell and Molecular Biology. 2011;**45**(2):189-201

[33] Holt PG, Strickland DH, Wikstrom ME, Jahnsen FL. Regulation of immunological homeostasis in the respiratory tract. Nature Reviews. Immunology. 2008;**8**(2):142-152

[34] Self WH, Courtney DM, McNaughton CD, Wunderink RG, Kline JA. High discordance of chest x-ray and computed tomography for detection of pulmonary opacities in ED patients: Implications for diagnosing pneumonia. The American Journal of Emergency Medicine. 2013;**31**(2):401-405

[35] Chavez MA, Shams N, Ellington LE, Naithani N, Gilman RH, Steinhoff MC,

et al. Lung ultrasound for the diagnosis of pneumonia in adults: A systematic review and meta-analysis. Respiratory Research. 2014;**15**:50

[36] Zheng N, Zhu D, Han Y. Procalcitonin and C-reactive protein perform better than the neutrophil/lymphocyte count ratio in evaluating hospital acquired pneumonia. BMC Pulmonary Medicine. 2020;**20**(1):166

[37] Fiori B, D'Inzeo T, Giaquinto A, Menchinelli G, Liotti FM, de Maio F, et al. Optimized use of the MALDI biotyper system and the filmarray BCID panel for direct identification of microbial pathogens from positive blood cultures. Journal of Clinical Microbiology. 2016;**54**(3):576-584

[38] Gastli N, Loubinoux J, Daragon M, Lavigne JP, Saint-Sardos P, Pailhories H, et al. Multicentric evaluation of biofire filmarray pneumonia panel for rapid bacteriological documentation of pneumonia. Clinical Microbiology and Infection. 2021;**27**(9):1308-1314

[39] Murphy CN, Fowler R, Balada-Llasat JM, Carroll A, Stone H, Akerele O, et al. Multicenter evaluation of the biofire filmarray pneumonia/pneumonia plus panel for detection and quantification of agents of lower respiratory tract infection. Journal of Clinical Microbiology. 2020;**58**(7):1

[40] Buchan BW, Windham S, Balada-Llasat JM, Leber A, Harrington A, Relich R, et al. Practical comparison of the biofire filmarray pneumonia panel to routine diagnostic methods and potential impact on antimicrobial stewardship in adult hospitalized patients with lower respiratory tract infections. Journal of Clinical Microbiology. 2020;**58**(7):1-2

[41] Ranzani OT, De Pascale G, Park M. Diagnosis of nonventilated hospital-acquired pneumonia: How much do we

know? Current Opinion in Critical Care. 2018;**24**(5):339-346

[42] Garnier M, Rozencwajg S, Pham T, Vimont S, Blayau C, Hafiani M, et al. Evaluation of early antimicrobial therapy adaptation guided by the BetaLACTA(R) test: A case-control study. Critical Care. 2017;**21**(1):161

[43] Laurent T, Huang TD, Bogaerts P, Glupczynski Y. Evaluation of the betaLACTA test, a novel commercial chromogenic test for rapid detection of ceftazidime-nonsusceptible *pseudomonas aeruginosa* isolates. Journal of Clinical Microbiology. 2013;**51**(6): 1951-1954

[44] Garnier M, Gallah S, Vimont S, Benzerara Y, Labbe V, Constant AL, et al. Multicentre randomised controlled trial to investigate usefulness of the rapid diagnostic betaLACTA test performed directly on bacterial cell pellets from respiratory, urinary or blood samples for the early de-escalation of carbapenems in septic intensive care unit patients: The BLUE-CarbA protocol. BMJ Open. 2019;**9**(2): e024561

[45] American Thoracic Society, Infectious Diseases Society of America. Guidelines for the management of adults with hospital-acquired, ventilator-associated, and healthcare-associated pneumonia. American Journal of Respiratory and Critical Care Medicine. 2005;**171**(4):388-416

[46] Stevens JP, Silva G, Gillis J, Novack V, Talmor D, Klompas M, et al. Automated surveillance for ventilator-associated events. Chest. 2014;**146**(6): 1612-1618

[47] Tumbarello M, De Pascale G, Trecarichi EM, Spanu T, Antonicelli F, Maviglia R, et al. Clinical outcomes of *pseudomonas aeruginosa* pneumonia in intensive care unit patients. Intensive Care Medicine. 2013;**39**(4):682-692

[48] De Bus L, Saerens L, Gadeyne B, Boelens J, Claeys G, De Waele JJ, et al. Development of antibiotic treatment algorithms based on local ecology and respiratory surveillance cultures to restrict the use of broad-spectrum antimicrobial drugs in the treatment of hospital-acquired pneumonia in the intensive care unit: A retrospective analysis. Critical Care. 2014;**18**(4):R152

[49] Di Pasquale M, Ferrer M, Esperatti M, Crisafulli E, Giunta V, Li Bassi G, et al. Assessment of severity of ICU-acquired pneumonia and association with etiology. Critical Care Medicine. 2014;**42**(2):303-312

[50] Mergenhagen KA, Starr KE, Wattengel BA, Lesse AJ, Sumon Z, Sellick JA. Determining the utility of methicillin-resistant staphylococcus aureus nares screening in antimicrobial stewardship. Clinical Infectious Diseases. 2020;**71**(5):1142-1148

[51] Haidar G, Philips NJ, Shields RK, Snyder D, Cheng S, Potoski BA, et al. Ceftolozane-tazobactam for the treatment of multidrug-resistant *pseudomonas aeruginosa* infections: Clinical effectiveness and evolution of resistance. Clinical Infectious Diseases. 2017;**65**(1):110-120

[52] Chastre J, Wolff M, Fagon JY, Chevret S, Thomas F, Wermert D, et al. Comparison of 8 vs 15 days of antibiotic therapy for ventilator-associated pneumonia in adults: A randomized trial. Journal of the American Medical Association. 2003; **290**(19):2588-2598

[53] Que Y-A, Moreillon P. 196— *Staphylococcus aureus* (Including staphylococcal toxic shock syndrome). In: Bennett JE, Dolin R, Blaser MJ, editors. Mandell, Douglas, and Bennett's Principles and Practice of Infectious Diseases (Eighth Edition). Philadelphia: W.B. Saunders; 2015. pp. 2237-71.e5

[54] Lyons PG, Kollef MH. Prevention of hospital-acquired pneumonia. Current Opinion in Critical Care. 2018;**24**(5): 370-378

[55] Churpek MM, Snyder A, Han X, Sokol S, Pettit N, Howell MD, et al. Quick sepsis-related organ failure assessment, systemic inflammatory response syndrome, and early warning scores for detecting clinical deterioration in infected patients outside the intensive care unit. American Journal of Respiratory and Critical Care Medicine. 2017;**195**(7): 906-911

[56] Burton LA, Price R, Barr KE, McAuley SM, Allen JB, Clinton AM, et al. Hospital-acquired pneumonia incidence and diagnosis in older patients. Age and Ageing. 2016;**45**(1): 171-174

[57] Boyce JM, Pittet D. Healthcare infection control practices advisory C, Force HSAIHHT. Guideline for hand hygiene in health-care settings. Recommendations of the healthcare infection control practices advisory committee and the HICPAC/SHEA/ APIC/IDSA hand hygiene task force. Society for healthcare epidemiology of America/Association for professionals in infection control/Infectious diseases society of America. MMWR Recommendations Report. 2002;**51** (RR-16):1-45

[58] O'Flaherty N, Fenelon L. The stethoscope and healthcare-associated infection: A snake in the grass or innocent bystander? The Journal of Hospital Infection. 2015;**91**(1):1-7

[59] Alvarez JA, Ruiz SR, Mosqueda JL, Leon X, Arreguin V, Macias AE, et al. Decontamination of stethoscope membranes with chlorhexidine: Should it be recommended? American Journal of Infection Control. 2016;**44**(11): e205-e2e9

[60] Maki DG. Stethoscopes and health care-associated infection. Mayo Clinic Proceedings. 2014;**89**(3):277-280

[61] Whitby M, Pessoa-Silva CL, McLaws ML, Allegranzi B, Sax H, Larson E, et al. Behavioural considerations for hand hygiene practices: The basic building blocks. The Journal of Hospital Infection. 2007; **65**(1):1-8

[62] Harris AD, Pineles L, Belton B, Johnson JK, Shardell M, Loeb M, et al. Universal glove and gown use and acquisition of antibiotic-resistant bacteria in the ICU: A randomized trial. Journal of the American Medical Association. 2013;**310**(15):1571-1580

[63] Nelson RE, Jones M, Leecaster M, Samore MH, Ray W, Huttner A, et al. An Economic analysis of strategies to control clostridium difficile transmission and infection using an agent-based simulation model. PLoS One. 2016;**11**(3):e0152248

[64] Saito T, Oobayashi K, Shimazaki Y, Yamashita Y, Iwasa Y, Nabeshima F, et al. Association of dry tongue to pyrexia in long-term hospitalized patients. Gerontology. 2008;**54**(2):87-91

[65] Riley P, Glenny AM, Hua F, Worthington HV. Pharmacological interventions for preventing dry mouth and salivary gland dysfunction following radiotherapy. Cochrane Database of Systematic Reviews. 2017;7: CD012744

[66] Titsworth WL, Abram J, Fullerton A, Hester J, Guin P, Waters MF, et al. Prospective quality initiative to maximize dysphagia screening reduces hospital-acquired pneumonia prevalence in patients with stroke. Stroke. 2013;**44**(11):3154-3160

[67] Ebihara T, Ebihara S, Yamazaki M, Asada M, Yamanda S, Arai H. Intensive stepwise method for oral intake using a

combination of transient receptor potential stimulation and olfactory stimulation inhibits the incidence of pneumonia in dysphagic older adults. Journal of the American Geriatrics Society. 2010;**58**(1):196-198

[68] Alhazzani W, Almasoud A, Jaeschke R, Lo BW, Sindi A, Altayyar S, et al. Small bowel feeding and risk of pneumonia in adult critically ill patients: A systematic review and meta-analysis of randomized trials. Critical Care. 2013; **17**(4):R127

[69] Liu Y, Dong X, Yang S, Wang A, Wang M. Metoclopramide for preventing nosocomial pneumonia in patients fed via nasogastric tubes: A systematic review and meta-analysis of randomized controlled trials. Asia Pacific Journal of Clinical Nutrition. 2017;**26**(5):820-828

[70] Wang L, Li X, Yang Z, Tang X, Yuan Q, Deng L, et al. Semi-recumbent position versus supine position for the prevention of ventilator-associated pneumonia in adults requiring mechanical ventilation. Cochrane Database of Systematic Reviews. 2016;**1**: CD009946

[71] Stolbrink M, McGowan L, Saman H, Nguyen T, Knightly R, Sharpe J, et al. The Early Mobility Bundle: A simple enhancement of therapy which may reduce incidence of hospital-acquired pneumonia and length of hospital stay. The Journal of Hospital Infection. 2014; **88**(1):34-39

[72] Cuesy PG, Sotomayor PL, Pina JO. Reduction in the incidence of poststroke nosocomial pneumonia by using the "turn-mob" program. Journal of Stroke and Cerebrovascular Diseases. 2010; **19**(1):23-28

[73] Scannapieco FA, Bush RB, Paju S. Associations between periodontal disease and risk for nosocomial bacterial pneumonia and chronic obstructive pulmonary disease. A systematic review. Annals of Periodontology. 2003;**8**(1): 54-69

[74] Watando A, Ebihara S, Ebihara T, Okazaki T, Takahashi H, Asada M, et al. Daily oral care and cough reflex sensitivity in elderly nursing home patients. Chest. 2004;**126**(4):1066-1070

[75] Nakajoh K, Nakagawa T, Sekizawa K, Matsui T, Arai H, Sasaki H. Relation between incidence of pneumonia and protective reflexes in post-stroke patients with oral or tube feeding. Journal of Internal Medicine. 2000;**247**(1):39-42

[76] El-Rabbany M, Zaghlol N, Bhandari M, Azarpazhooh A. Prophylactic oral health procedures to prevent hospital-acquired and ventilator-associated pneumonia: A systematic review. International Journal of Nursing Studies. 2015;**52**(1):452-464

[77] Swan JT, Ashton CM, Bui LN, Pham VP, Shirkey BA, Blackshear JE, et al. Effect of chlorhexidine bathing every other day on prevention of hospital-acquired infections in the surgical ICU: A single-center, randomized controlled trial. Critical Care Medicine. 2016;**44**(10):1822-1832

[78] Klompas M, Speck K, Howell MD, Greene LR, Berenholtz SM. Reappraisal of routine oral care with chlorhexidine gluconate for patients receiving mechanical ventilation: Systematic review and meta-analysis. JAMA Internal Medicine. 2014;**174**(5):751-761

[79] Roquilly A, Marret E, Abraham E, Asehnoune K. Pneumonia prevention to decrease mortality in intensive care unit: A systematic review and meta-analysis. Clinical Infectious Diseases. 2015;**60**(1): 64-75

[80] Shinefield H, Black S, Fattom A, Horwith G, Rasgon S, Ordonez J, et al. Use of a Staphylococcus aureus

conjugate vaccine in patients receiving hemodialysis. The New England Journal of Medicine. 2002;**346**(7):491-496

[81] Francois B, Luyt CE, Dugard A, Wolff M, Diehl JL, Jaber S, et al. Safety and pharmacokinetics of an anti-PcrV PEGylated monoclonal antibody fragment in mechanically ventilated patients colonized with *Pseudomonas aeruginosa*: A randomized,double-blind, placebo-controlled trial. Critical Care Medicine. 2012;**40**(8):2320-2326

[82] Herzig SJ, Howell MD, Ngo LH, Marcantonio ER. Acid-suppressive medication use and the risk for hospital-acquired pneumonia. Journal of the American Medical Association. 2009; **301**(20):2120-2128

[83] Gill SK, Hui K, Farne H, Garnett JP, Baines DL, Moore LS, et al. Increased airway glucose increases airway bacterial load in hyperglycaemia. Scientific Reports. 2016;**6**:27636

[84] Garnett JP, Baker EH, Baines DL. Sweet talk: Insights into the nature and importance of glucose transport in lung epithelium. The European Respiratory Journal. 2012;**40**(5):1269-1276

[85] Yang M, Yan Y, Yin X, Wang BY, Wu T, Liu GJ, et al. Chest physiotherapy for pneumonia in adults. Cochrane Database of Systematic Reviews. 2013;**2**: CD006338

[86] Pasquina P, Tramer MR, Granier JM, Walder B. Respiratory physiotherapy to prevent pulmonary complications after abdominal surgery: A systematic review. Chest. 2006; **130**(6):1887-1899

[87] Girou E, Schortgen F, Delclaux C, Brun-Buisson C, Blot F, Lefort Y, et al. Association of noninvasive ventilation with nosocomial infections and survival in critically ill patients. Journal of the American Medical Association. 2000; **284**(18):2361-2367

[88] Stephan F, Barrucand B, Petit P, Rezaiguia-Delclaux S, Medard A, Delannoy B, et al. High-flow nasal oxygen vs noninvasive positive airway pressure in hypoxemic patients after cardiothoracic surgery: A randomized clinical trial. Journal of the American Medical Association. 2015;**313**(23): 2331-2339

[89] Frat JP, Thille AW, Mercat A, Girault C, Ragot S, Perbet S, et al. High-flow oxygen through nasal cannula in acute hypoxemic respiratory failure. The New England Journal of Medicine. 2015;**372**(23):2185-2196

[90] Rocco M, Dell'Utri D, Morelli A, Spadetta G, Conti G, Antonelli M, et al. Noninvasive ventilation by helmet or face mask in immunocompromised patients: A case-control study. Chest. 2004;**126**(5):1508-1515

[91] Kane RL, Shamliyan TA, Mueller C, Duval S, Wilt TJ. The association of registered nurse staffing levels and patient outcomes: Systematic review and meta-analysis. Medical Care. 2007; **45**(12):1195-1204

[92] Wilcox ME, Chong CA, Niven DJ, Rubenfeld GD, Rowan KM, Wunsch H, et al. Do intensivist staffing patterns influence hospital mortality following ICU admission? A systematic review and meta-analyses. Critical Care Medicine. 2013;**41**(10):2253-2274

Chapter 3

Pneumonia: Drug-Related Problems and Hospital Readmissions

Kien T. Nguyen, Suol T. Pham, Thu P.M. Vo, Chu X. Duong,
Dyah A. Perwitasari, Ngoc H.K. Truong, Dung T.H. Quach,
Thao N.P. Nguyen, Van T.T. Duong, Phuong M. Nguyen,
Thao H. Nguyen, Katja Taxis and Thang Nguyen

Abstract

Pneumonia is one of the most common infectious diseases and the fourth leading cause of death globally. According to US statistics in 2019, pneumonia is the most common cause of sepsis and septic shock. In the US, inpatient pneumonia hospitalizations account for the top 10 highest medical costs, totaling $9.5 billion for 960,000 hospital stays. The emergence of antibiotic resistance in the treatment of infectious diseases, including the treatment of pneumonia, is a globally alarming problem. Antibiotic resistance increases the risk of death and re-hospitalization, prolongs hospital stays, and increases treatment costs, and is one of the greatest threats in modern medicine. Drug-related problems (DRPs) in pneumonia - such as suboptimal antibiotic indications, prolonged treatment duration, and drug interactions - increase the rate of antibiotic resistance and adverse effects, thereby leading to an increased burden in treatment. In a context in which novel and effective antibiotics are scarce, mitigating DRPs in order to reduce antibiotic resistance is currently a prime concern. A variety of interventions proven useful in reducing DRPs are antibiotic stewardship programs, the use of biomarkers, computerized physician order entries and clinical decision support systems, and community-acquired pneumonia scores.

Keywords: Pneumonia, drug-related problems, re-hospitalization, prescriptions, interventions

1. Introduction

Pneumonia is an acute lower respiratory tract infection caused by bacteria, viruses, or fungi. Groups of patients at high risk of getting pneumonia include children under 5 years old, people over 65 years old, and people with comorbidities. Pneumonia is the leading cause of death in children, and among the top four causes of death globally [1]. Each year, pneumonia kills more than 800,000 children under the age of 5, equivalent to about 2,200 children every day [2]. In the United States, the annual incidence of community-acquired pneumonia (CAP) was 248 cases per 100,000 persons [3]. A study in central Vietnam reported that the incidence of CAP in subjects aged ≥ 65 years was 4.6 per 1,000 person-years (95% CI, 3.8–5.5) [4]. Hospitalized patients diagnosed with pneumonia accounted for 19.9%, 6.4%, and 1.5% in the Philippines, Malaysia, and Indonesia, respectively. The total estimated costs incurred for pneumonia patients were in Malaysia 4.1 million USD, in Indonesia 2.6 million USD, and in the Philippines 2.6 million USD [5].

Drug-related problems are defined as 'events or circumstances involving drug therapy that actually or potentially interfere with desired health outcomes' [6]. Causes of DRPs can be related to inappropriate drug selection, inappropriate dosage, duration of use of medication longer or shorter than recommended, incorrect drug use processes, or poor compliance, all resulting in decreased treatment effectiveness and increased morbidity and mortality [7–9]. In Ethiopia, the proportion of patients hospitalized for infectious diseases, and who also had DRPs, was 71.51% (123/172); of these, the unnecessary broad-spectrum antibiotic option ceftriaxone accounted for 44.77% [10]. Similarly, in a study in Spain, almost half (45.1%) of hospitalized patients suffered from DRPs [11]. Common DRPs associated with pneumonia include inappropriate antibiotic indications, prolonged antibiotic treatment, and overtreatment, which may lead to potential drug–drug interactions [12–15]. In the context of increasing antibiotic resistance, prescribing doctors, often concerned about possibly missing pathogenic bacteria, tend to prescribe broad-spectrum antibiotics over a longer treatment time to avoid recurrence of the disease. Fear, rather than lack of knowledge, is a major barrier to preventing overtreatment with antibiotics [16]. Therefore, a new method being considered for improving empirical antibiotic selection is the community-acquired pneumonia score. This score can be used in a prediction model of clinical data, enabling more accurate application of empirical antibiotics [17]. In addition, many intervention tools need to be applied, such as antibiotic management programs, biomarkers, and computerized physician order entries (CPOE), to ensure the effectiveness and safety of guideline compliance. The computerized physician order entry (CPOE) and clinical decision support systems (CDSS) are valuable technological tools for use in interventions to prevent adverse drug events (ADEs). However, in the healthcare system, the role of the clinical pharmacist in minimizing DRPs remains crucial [14]. The chapter is, therefore, to summarize an overview of DRPs in pneumonia and recommend some strategies for reducing these DRPs.

2. Drug-related problems in pneumonia

2.1 Improper drug selection and dose selection

Prescribing inappropriate antibiotics leads to increased mortality, the development of antimicrobial resistance, and added treatment costs [18, 19]. Meta-analysis of 7401 patients with ventilator-associated pneumonia (VAP), using unadjusted data, revealed that inappropriate antibiotic therapy significantly increased the mortality of patients (odds ratio [OR], 2.34; 95% CI, 1.51–3.63; P = 0.0001, I2 = 28.5%) [8]. A retrospective cohort study of bacteremic pneumonia, conducted in Barnes-Jewish Hospital in Missouri, USA (2008–2015) using multivariable logistic regression analysis for hospital mortality, indicated that inappropriate initial antibiotic treatment had the greatest odds ratio with mortality (OR 2.2, 95% CI 1.5–3.2, P < 0.001). The rate of inappropriate antibiotic initiation was significantly higher in patients with ceftriaxone-resistant pathogens than with ceftriaxone-susceptible pathogens (27.9% vs. 7.1%, P < 0.001), and the associated hospital mortality rates were respectively 41.5% vs. 32.0% (P = 0.001) [9].

Inappropriate antibiotic selection is one of the most common DRPs in patients with pneumonia, and particularly community-acquired pneumonia (CAP). Antibiotic prescriptions collected from 22 pharmacies in Mongolia indicated that inappropriate drug selection affected both adults (57.7%) and children (56.6%) [20]. A study among 518 outpatients with CAP in the Veterans Affairs Western New York Healthcare System indicated that 69% of patients received an inappropriate antibiotic; for 76.7% of them an incorrect drug had been prescribed, based on the patient's comorbidities [21]. In Thailand, a prospective observational study of severe CAP in general medical wards showed that 52% of patients received initial antibiotic regimens that were discordant with IDSA/ATS guidelines [22].

The increase in resistance rates of bacteria to antibiotics leads to inappropriate selection of initial antibiotics. Due to an "encirclement" mentality, doctors often tend to choose empiric broad-spectrum antibiotics; this invisible cause increases antibiotic resistance, resulting in a "vicious circle" that increasingly burdens patients and society [23–25]. In particular, prescribing broad-spectrum antibiotics for a low-risk group increases the risk of unwanted effects rather than making treatment beneficial. According to current guidelines for the treatment of community-acquired pneumonia, an outpatient should receive beta-lactam or a macrolide or doxycycline [26, 27]. A retrospective chart review at a large hospital indicated that fluoroquinolones were antibiotics overprescribed for 71% of patients in the low-risk group [28]. Another retrospective chart review among 156 adult patients with a diagnosis of CAP, admitted to a community hospital emergency department in Canada, found that physicians overprescribed fluoroquinolones for 80.8% of patients who did not need them [29]. Over-prescribing of fluoroquinolones for outpatients with pneumonia increases the risk of side effects: tendon rupture, tendonitis, feeling shaky, unusual hunger, serious events of aortic ruptures or tears, and development of antibiotic resistance [30–32].

For this reason, antibiotic stewardship programs (ASPs) and clinical pharmacists play an important role in promoting the appropriate prescribing of empiric antibiotics. A retrospective cohort study of patients with CAP indicated a significant reduction in fluoroquinolone prescribing over time following intervention involving ASPs and clinical pharmacists [33]. An additional new method for improving empirical antibiotic selection is the community-acquired pneumonia score. This score provides a model of clinical data, thereby enabling the proper use of empirical antibiotics [17]. Implementation of an empiric therapy guide is important to minimize DRPs in the initial selection of antibiotics for pneumonia, as the causative organism and the patient's susceptibility to it are often unknown at the time of prescription. Galanter KM et al. demonstrated that after intervention in accordance with the empiric therapy guide, the rate of broad-spectrum antibiotic indication for CAP decreased significantly, by 17.0% [34].

In Canada, a study on pneumonia showed that prescribed antibiotic doses tended to be higher than recommended [29]. In contrast, a prospective multinational study involving 68 ICUs across 10 countries confirmed that 20% of patients received less than the most conservative PK/PD target (50% f T > MIC), and fewer than 50% of patients received a preferred PK/PD target (100% f T > MIC) [13]. Such insufficient antibiotic exposure can also facilitate antibiotic resistance. For the treatment of CAP, especially critical patients require individualized dosing based on the severity of disease, local documented pathogen susceptibilities, and causal bacteria. Patient characteristics also play an important role in reducing mortality.

2.2 Drug interactions

Pneumonia patients often have not just one diagnosis but suffer from comorbid conditions. Frequent comorbidities are diabetes mellitus, cerebrovascular disease, chronic lung disease, chronic kidney disease, and dementia [15, 35, 36]. Common medication classes used for the management of comorbid conditions are cardio-vascular agents, alimentary tract and metabolism agents, nervous system agents, respiratory agents, blood-forming agents, and general anti-infective agents for sys-temic use. The potential of drug–drug interactions in cases of pneumonia is more prevalent in older patients, possibly leading to chronic diseases and polypharmacy; some drugs even increase the risks of pneumonia [37]. In pneumonia patients, comorbidities have been strongly associated with long-term mortality [36], and concurrent use of multiple drugs can lead to an increased risk of drug–drug interac-tions (DDIs) [15, 35, 38]. Results of a study in a population, most of whom were concurrently using >10 drugs, revealed that 73.1% of these patients faced potential DDIs. Indeed, more than half of the patients presented with major potential DDIs [15]. Furthermore, nearly 75% of patients with community-acquired pneumonia (CAP) were subjected to polypharmacy [35].

Some clinical consequences of DDIs included increased or decreased therapeutic effectiveness, adverse drug reactions (ADRs), and toxicity (nephrotoxicity, hepa-totoxicity) [15, 38]. DDIs can take place between different antibiotics, and between antibiotics and other medications. For treating pneumonia many guidelines recommend using β-lactams, macrolides, and fluoroquinolones. This may cause a prolonged QT interval (when fluoroquinolones or macrolides are administered) or a prolonged Prothrombin Time and International Normalized Ratio (INR) (if fluoroquinolones and warfarin are administered concurrently) [37]. Therefore, to prevent the negative effects of polypharmacy, consultations should be held to identify potential DDIs and alert physicians. Moreover, medical staff should refer to more than one drug interaction checker tool -- like Lexi-Interact, Micromedex, Medscape, Drugs.com. -- as well as adhere to guidelines for optimizing the use of prescribed drugs and discontinuing the use of unnecessary drugs.

2.3 Initiation and duration of administration antibiotic treatment

Patients whose initial appropriate antibiotics therapy is delayed may have increased morbidity rates compared to those receiving appropriately prescribed therapy on time. A systematic review in patients hospitalized with infections due to *Klebsiella pneumoniae* or *Escherichia coli* found that a delay in appropriate antibiotic therapy of more than 24 hours and 48 hours after culture collection, or in culture and susceptibility reporting, can increase the risk of mortality: OR 1.60 (95% CI, 1.25–2.50) and OR 1.76 (95% CI, 1.27–2.44) respectively [39]. A prospective cohort study in patients with VAP showed that for thirty-three patients (30.8%) the appropriate antibiotic treatment was delayed for >24 hours after they first met the diagnostic criteria for VAP; this initially delayed appropriate antibiotic treatment was a risk factor for increasing the hospital mortality rate (adjusted odds ratio, 7.68; 95% CI 4.50 to 13.09; p < 0.001) [40].

The British Thoracic Society Guidelines for the Management of Community-Acquired Pneumonia in Adults recommends the administration of antibiotics within four hours of admission to hospital for adults with radiologically confirmed CAP [41]. A large study (n = 13,725 from 188 institutions) conducted among adults hospitalized with CAP indicated that 37% of patients failed to receive antibiotics within four hours of admission. Delay time of the first antibiotic was associated with a greater OR of 30-day inpatient mortality. The adjusted 30-day inpatient mortality was lower for adults who received their initial antibiotic within four hours, compared with >4 hours (adjusted OR 0.84, 95% CI 0.74 to 0.94; p = 0.003) [42]. A retrospective study (n = 18,209) of Medicare patients older than 65 years who were hospitalized with CAP revealed that 39.1% did not receive antibiotics within four hours of admission. Initial administration of antibiotics within four hours, versus more than four hours, after arrival at the hospital was associated with reduced in-hospital mortality (6.8% vs. 7.4%; adjusted odds ratio (AOR)), 0.85; 95% CI, 0.74–0.98), versus mortality within 30 days of admission (11.6% vs. 12.7%; AOR, 0.85; 95% CI, 0.76–0.95), and length of stay exceeding the 5-day median (42.1% vs. 45.1%; AOR, 0.90; 95% CI, 0.83–0.96) [43].

For a long time, a seven-day application of antibiotic therapy to treat infectious diseases was standard procedure [44]. However, the duration of antibiotic treatment should be based on the severity of the disease, patient characteristics, patients' clinical stability, and the causative organisms [45]. Long-term antibiotic treatment is associated with increased side- effects, antibiotic-resistant organisms, and *C. difficile* diarrhea [46, 47]. Unfortunately, a large study in 66,901 long-term care residents showed that 44.9% of patients were prescribed antibiotic treatment lasting longer than 7 days, and prescriptions tended not to be based on patient characteristics and comorbidities [14]. Furthermore, a retrospective cohort of 152,874 patients hospitalized for CAP found that more than 70% were prescribed antibiotics in excess of recommendations [48]. A large US study found that for 93% and 71% of patients with uncomplicated CAP and healthcare-associated pneumonia, respectively, lengthy durations of antibiotic treatment were indicated [49].

In addition, a systematic review of HAP in critically ill adults (including VAP) manifested that a short duration of antibiotic therapy (7 to 8 days) versus conventional antibiotic therapy (10 to 15 days) did not increase mortality rate, duration of mechanical ventilation, and length of hospital stay; however, a rise in recurrence was discovered in the subgroup of patients with VAP, caused by non-fermenting Gram-negative bacilli [50]. An RCT study in neonatal pneumonia conducted to compare the efficacy of a short course (4 days, intervention group) with a traditional antibiotic regimen (7 days, control group) demonstrated that treatment in the intervention group had the same success rate as in the control group, but the group intervention significantly reduced the length of the hospital stay, as well as antibiotic use and treatment costs [51].

For adults with CAP, although more relevant antibiotic studies are needed in the future to support a short-term therapy, clinicians should always be aware that the duration of antibiotic treatment should be based on the clinical improvement of the patient rather than mechanical practice. ATS/IDSA guidelines recommend a total duration of antibiotic therapy of 5 days for most outpatients and inpatients with CAP, except for cases of suspected *MRSA* or *P. aeruginosa*. According to the guidelines, the patient will achieve clinical improvement after the first 48–72 hours, after which antibiotics should be continued for 2–3 days [45]. Pending further studies, adherence to guidelines is one of the keys to limiting DRPs in treatment.

For pediatric patients with CAP, according to the 2011 PIDS/IDSA guidelines, which are still applicable today, the duration of treatment depends upon the severity. Treatment courses of 10 days are recommended, although the guidelines suggest that shorter courses may be just as effective, especially in mild patients. CA-MRSA patients may need a longer treatment period [26].

For adults with HAP/VAP, although the duration of antibiotic use is determined based on patients' conditions like a clinical improvement, as well as radiological and laboratory parameters, the current recommendation for most patients is a 7-day course of antimicrobial therapy rather than longer treatment [52].

In conclusion, the high rate of prolongation of antibiotic treatment and inappropriate initiation of therapy in patients with pneumonia indicates the great need for improvement to reduce drug-related problems. Antimicrobial stewardship, biomarkers, and clinical stability scores should be applied to decrease the duration of antibiotic therapy [53, 54].

2.4 Comorbidities

Respiratory diseases have been found to be associated with multi-morbidity patterns [55]. Patients with pneumonia often have a broad range of comorbid conditions [37, 56]. While short-term mortality is directly associated with the severity of pneumonia, long-term mortality is associated with comorbid conditions [56]. Most patients who die from pneumonia have one or more severe chronic diseases, such as cerebrovascular disease, chronic cardiac or renal disease, dementia, cachexia, mobility impairment, neoplastic metastatic disease, or sepsis. Patients with either MRSA or Pseudomonas were found to have an increased risk of dying of pneumonia [57]. In patients with pneumonia, comorbidities are also associated with poor response to treatment. Moreover, patients older than 80 years with comorbidities also have a higher mortality rate than patients from other age groups [58].

All-cause mortality has been found to increase in relation to the number of comorbid conditions. Every comorbid condition has been found to correlate with a 9% higher risk of death [56]. Some comorbid conditions that influence mortality (cardiovascular and lung diseases, diabetes, etc.) are also particular risk factors for pneumonia [37].

The Charlson Comorbidity Index measures comorbidity. Patients with a higher Charlson pathology index score were found to have a higher risk of death due to hospitalization (OR 1.28; 95% CI 1.07–1.53). These findings indicate a relationship between a patient's comorbid burden and the consequences of community-acquired pneumonia [59]. Results of a study among 108 patients by Franzen et al. indicated that the death risk of hospitalized pneumonia patients tended to increase with a higher CCI [58].

Children with comorbidities were more likely to be hospitalized for community-acquired pneumonia, compared to those without comorbidities. Approximately 50% of children and adolescents with community-acquired pneumonia had comorbidities related to malnutrition, as well as the use of antibiotics and hospitalization for community-acquired pneumonia during the previous 24 months. Bivariate analysis showed that patients with comorbidities demonstrated higher chances of malnutrition (p = 0.002), previous use of antibiotics (p = 0.008), and previous hospitalization for community-acquired pneumonia in the last 24 months (p = 0.004). In multivariate analysis, the following variables were independent predictors of community-acquired pneumonia in patients with comorbidities: malnutrition (p = 0.008; RR = 1.75; 95%CI 1.75–44.60); previous use of antibiotics (p = 0.0013; RR = 3.03; 95%CI 1.27–7.20); and previous hospitalization for community-acquired pneumonia (p = 0.035; RR = 2.91; 95%CI 1.08–7.90) [60].

In addition, pneumonia influenced concurrent comorbid conditions, resulting in a subsequent impact on the incidence of events like acute myocardial infarction, heart failure, stroke, venous thromboembolism, and cancer [56]. Recognition of the mutual relationship between pneumonia and comorbidities will help to identify patients at high risk. Though no specific guideline for multi-morbidities currently exists, close monitoring of patients during hospitalization and long-term follow-up may result in better outcomes.

2.5 Risk factors for DRP-readmission and pneumonia re-hospitalization

According to a review on drug-related hospital readmissions, an average of 21% of such readmissions were drug-related, and 69% were considered preventable [61]. Some predictive factors that can be considered to avoid hospital readmissions due to DRPs include limiting the number of drugs prescribed on a particular day, and the number of drug classifications according to the day of hospitalization [62]. Healthcare professionals should focus more on identifying risk factors related to drug-related readmissions, and on finding appropriate interventions.

Among the known risk factors for DRPs is non-adherence to medication, which may be aggravated by the complexity of the medication regimen. The medication regimen complexity index (MRCI) is a tool that assesses the complexity of a medication list in terms of dosage form, dosing frequency, and additional directions required for administration. Higher MRCI scores indicate greater regimen complexity. MRCI scores were significantly higher in patients readmitted (within 30 days) than those not readmitted [63, 64]. The MRCI can thus be used as a predictor of drug-related readmissions.

Another risk factor associated with 30-day readmission rates was the presence of comorbidities [65]. Comorbidities weaken the immune system and worsen a patient's condition. The Charlson Comorbidity Index (CCI) is a tool that adds weighted scores to each illness predictive of mortality. Some studies have reported a higher mean CCI in patients who were re-admitted [62, 65]. As the CCI apparently has a strong potential to be a readmission predictor, it has been recommended for inclusion in readmission prediction tools [63].

Risk factors for pneumonia re-hospitalization are currently among the most important problems to be dealt with. Possible risk factors for early re-hospitalizations include male gender, age ≥70 years, the longer length of stay during the first admission, and a Multisource Comorbidity Score (MCS) ≥10. As for therapy, for readmitted CAP patients whose underlying respiratory disease has not yet been determined, the value of inhaled therapy has not definitely been decided. "Inhaled steroids may favor CAP in COPD patients, whereas anticholinergics may favor CAP in asthma patients. It is difficult to differentiate the effect of inhaled therapy from the effect of COPD or asthma severity on the risk of CAP, and these relationships may not be causal, but could call attention to inhaled therapy in COPD and asthma patients." [66]. In pediatric patients infected with Mycoplasma pneumonia, readmission before 90 days after discharge is influenced by age, body temperature, and *influenza A* co-infection during hospitalization [67]. However, in adult patients, risk factors for readmission within 30 days after hospital discharge include the person's age, hospitalization frequency during 3 months, chronic respiratory failure, heart failure, chronic liver disease, and the (non)availability of home healthcare [68].

A post-discharge study was performed in which researchers phoned every patient within 48–96 hours after they left the hospital to ask about their medication adherence, any adverse drug events (ADEs), and their use of medication. The process of medication reconciliation identified 103 errors, or 2.4 errors per patient, especially errors related to inaccurate doses, frequency, or medications not included on the list of home medications (**Table 1**) [69].

Multivariable analysis showed pneumonia-related readmission to be connected to para/hemiplegia, malignancy, pneumonia severity index class ≥4, and clinical instability ≥1 upon hospital discharge. Comorbidities such as chronic lung disease and chronic kidney disease, treatment failure, and decompensation of comorbidities were correlated with the pneumonia-unrelated 30-day re-hospitalization rate [65].

Interventions (n = 186)	n (%)
Medication reconciliation (n = 103)	
Incorrect dose or frequency	49 (48)
Medication omitted	33 (32)
Medication added	14 (14)
Duplicate therapy	4 (4)
Counseled in nonadherence	3 (3)
Mean errors per patient[a]	2.4
Therapeutic recommendations (n = 38)	
Change route	29 (76)
Optimize therapy	7 (18)
De-escalate therapy	2 (5)
Discharge counseling (n = 45)	
Counseling on antibiotics[b]	33 (73)
Counseling on chronic medication changes	12 (27)

Note: All data are given as n (%) unless otherwise specified, and all percentages are rounded to the nearest whole number.
[a]n = 43 patients.
[b]n = 39 patients were prescribed discharge antibiotics.

Table 1.
Medication errors identified, and pharmacist interventions.

3. Strategies for reducing DRPs in pneumonia

3.1 Role of a clinical hospital pharmacist in patient care

Various interventions are needed, focused on reducing the risk of hospital readmissions by choosing transitional and territorial care and synchronizing post-discharge care [66]. Pharmacist-bundled interference was associated with a decline in the 30-day readmission rate for high-risk patients with pneumonia. Consequently, reducing hospital readmissions by supplying the greatest possible quality of health care is now becoming an essential consideration, also for the institutions themselves [69]. Also, identifying drug-resistant pathogens in pneumonia patients may help to determine the appropriate choice of empirical antibiotics. Further, building a model to define the patient's risk factors may help with the prescription of broad-spectrum antibiotics [70]. Antibiotic administration for outpatients can be improved by predicting factors related to inappropriate antibiotic regimens. Patients at risk of drug resistance are now among the predictors of unsuitable antibiotic regimens [21].

The outcomes of this pilot research show that a pharmacist-specific bundled intervention, involving medication reconciliation, curative advice, patient discharge direction, and a research phone call, was associated with a decreased 30-day readmission rate for high-risk patients with pneumonia. The more than 200 total interventions reported suggest countless promising opportunities for increased pharmacist participation in care. Permitting pharmacists to devote time and effort to high-risk patient populations could confirm their value in supporting and expanding services to other people in the future, as well as reduce health care prices, and eventually the extent of welfare patient care [69].

Modifying the route of administration (ex- or intravenous to oral) was the most popular intervention, second to optimizing therapy. Optimizing therapy included making suitable renal doses and suggesting substitute regimens, especially if a patient's inpatient antibiotic regimen was the same as an outpatient regimen that had failed, or if he or she had risk factors for a healthcare-associated infection. Regarding the element of discharge counseling in the intervention, 91% of patients chosen prospectively for a pilot study received such counseling. This single-center pilot research concentrated on the influence pharmacists can have on transitions of care and readmission rates, using interventions like medication reconciliation, therapeutic recommendations, discharge instructions, and follow-up [66].

3.2 Antibiotic stewardship programs

J.E. McGowan Jr. and D.N. Gerding were the first to create the term "antimicrobial stewardship" in an article published in 1996. They wanted to emphasize the need for appropriate antibiotic prescription in order to prevent resistance [71]. IDSA defined these as "antibiotic stewardship programs referring to coordinated interventions designed to improve and measure the appropriate use of antimicrobial agents" [72]. The 5 "Rs" of anti-microbial stewardship are: "the right drug at the right time with the right dose for the right bug for the right duration" [16]. The goals of ASP increase treatment effectiveness while reducing *C. difficile* infections, adverse effects, antibiotic resistance, hospital costs, and lengths of stay. Some activities related to antibiotic stewardship in CAP include monitoring the de-escalation and duration of antibiotic treatment, complying with treatment guidelines, switching from intravenous to oral antibiotic treatments, prospective auditing, and developing the multidisciplinary team [73]. Antibiotic stewardship contributes to rational prescription of antibiotics, increases treatment effectiveness, and reduces side-effects and antibiotic resistance. A multi-center, pre-empirical, quasi-experimental study including 600 CAP patients (307 in the historical control group and 293 in the stewardship intervention group) showed that antibiotic stewardship helped to increase guideline-concordance to the duration of antibiotic therapy from 5.6% in the historical group to 42% in the intervention group (P = 0.001). The intervention group received a significantly shorter mean duration of treatment than the historical group (6 (5–7) versus 9 (7–10) days, P = 0.001). Antibiotic stewardship helped to avoid a total of 586 days of unnecessary antibiotics during the 6-month intervention period, while incidence of readmission for CAP, mortality rate within 30 days post-discharge were similar in both groups [54]. A multicenter randomized trial including 312 hospitalized CAP patients found that the duration of antibiotic therapy as determined by the physician (control group) was longer than in the guideline-concordant group (intervention group): (median, 10 days [interquartile range, 10–11]) versus 5 days (interquartile range, 5–6.5), respectively; P < .001). Clinical success was similar between both groups, at both 10 days (48.6% versus 56.3%) and 30 days (88.6% versus 91.9%) after admission [73].

The major activities and elements of ASPs include [74]:

- Hospital Leadership Commitment

- Accountability

- Pharmacy Expertise

- Action

- Tracking

- Reporting

- Education

Hospital Leadership Commitment: The senior leadership of the hospital, especially the chief medical officer, plays an important role in the success of ASPs. Hospital leadership helps to provide ASPs with the resources needed to achieve their goals.

Accountability: ASPs must have a designated leader or co-leaders, such as a physician and pharmacist, who have effective leadership, management, and communication skills, and are responsible for program management and outcomes.

Pharmacy Expertise: The participation of pharmacists, ideally as co-leaders of ASPs, will help to make ASPs highly effective. In large hospitals, pharmacists with infectious disease training are designated, but in hospitals without infectious disease trained pharmacists, general clinical pharmacists are appointed to help lead implementation efforts to improve antibiotic use.

Action: Antibiotic stewardship interventions are initiated to improve antibiotic use. Some activities related to antibiotic stewardship in CAP include prospective audit and feedback, such as monitoring the de-escalation and duration of antibiotic treatment, complying with treatment guidelines, switching from intravenous to oral antibiotic treatments, and preauthorization. The three priority interventions are: prospective audit and feedback, preauthorization, and facility-specific treatment guidelines.

- Preauthorization: This requires prescribers to gain approval prior to the use of certain antibiotics. This can help to optimize initial empiric therapy. The development of preauthorization for necessary antibiotics can be based on standard guidelines; limited antibiotics can be prescribed based on consultation, or more easily, referring to the WHO antibiotic classification. In 2017, WHO proposed categorizing antibiotics into three groups: ACCESS, WATCH, and RESERVE groups [75]. For the WATCH group, antibiotics with a high risk of resistance, such as 3rd-generation cephalosporins, carbapenems, and fluoroquinolones, should be preauthorized; for the RESERVE group, antibiotics such as colistin, ceftaroline, tigecycline, and aztreonam are indicated when other prescribed antibiotics have failed or are inadequate (e.g., serious life-threatening infections due to multidrug-resistant bacteria), and must be authorized and discussed before prescribing.

- Prospective audit and feedback: This is an external assessment of antibiotic therapy by ASP experts at some point after the agent has been prescribed. The ASP prospective audit and feedback team usually consists of a physician (an infectious disease specialist or a clinical microbiologist) and a clinical pharmacist. Prospective audit and feedback are performed as follows: On the first day of prescribed antibiotics, the team audits the suitability of doses and the routes of empirical antibiotic therapy. After 72 hours, the team reviews the patient's response (clinical stability, biomarkers, renal function), along with microbiological culture results, to give feedback to the treating physician in case a need to change the therapy is indicated: change of antibiotic, the addition of antibiotic, de-escalation of antibiotic treatment, dose adjustment. The cycle of audit and feedback is performed continuously. On day 7, the team evaluates the duration of antibiotic treatment (**Figure 1**) [76]. Preauthorization and

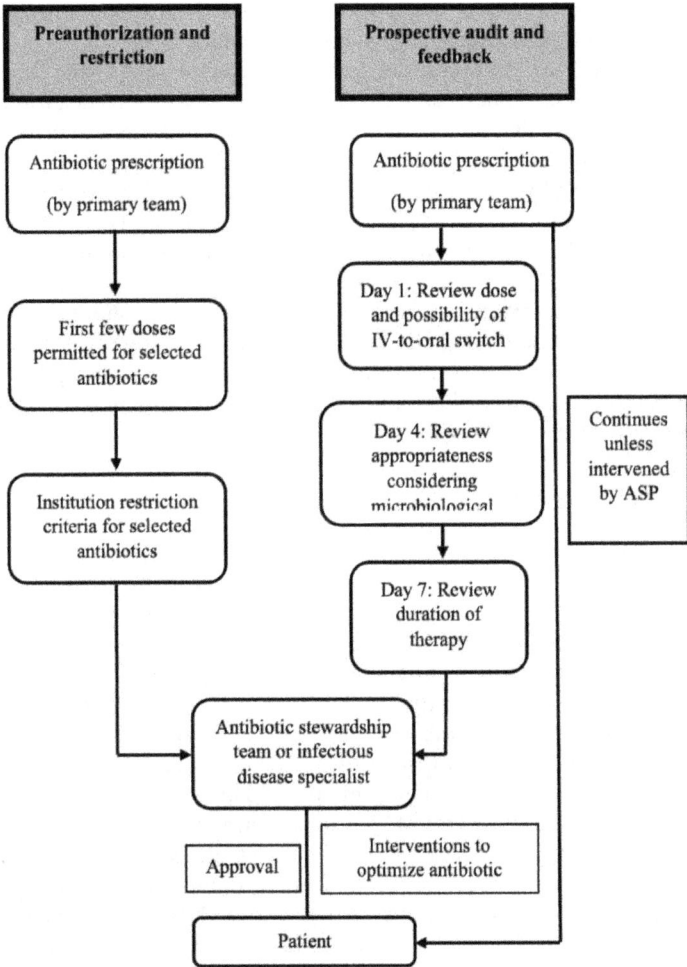

Figure 1.
Schema for prospective audit and feedback, and formulary restriction and preauthorization, for ASPs.

prospective audit and feedback are complementary processes that optimize antibiotic therapy. Preauthorization resembles an antibiotic input "filter" that improves initiation of antibiotics, and prospective audit and feedback help to optimize continued therapy.

- Facility-specific treatment guidelines: A clear guideline on antibiotic use will help to make prospective audit and feedback easier and more effective. Recommendations should be developed based on national and international guidelines, local susceptibilities, and hospital antibiotic management policies.

Tracking: Measurement is crucial to identify opportunities for improvement and to assess the impact of interventions. Measurement of antibiotic stewardship interventions may include measures of antibiotic use, and measures of outcomes like *C. difficile* infections, antibiotic resistance, and financial impact.

Reporting: A comprehensive picture of antibiotic use and antibiotic resistance, along with the work of the antibiotic stewardship program, should be provided in regular updates to prescribers, pharmacists, nurses, and leadership. This helps make medical staff aware of the situation of antibiotic use and antibiotic resistance at their facility, thereby promoting rational use of antibiotics.

Education: Interventions (preauthorization, prospective audit, and feedback) and measurement of antibiotic use and outcomes, can reveal gaps in antibiotic prescribing in hospitals. This helps to make the education of medical professionals realistic and effective, thereby gradually improving the effectiveness of antibiotic treatment, reducing adverse effects, antibiotic resistance, and treatment costs. There are many ways to provide education regarding antibiotic use, such as presentations; posters, flyers, and newsletters; and/or electronic communication to staff groups.

In summary, ASP interventions applied in hospitals, such as audit and feedback, updating of treatment guidelines along with local susceptibility patterns, and training of medical staff, can reveal individual or departmental cases of high antibiotic use by infectious disease specialists, clinical pharmacists, and microbiologists in order to promote rational antibiotic use [77].

3.3 Technological tools

3.3.1 Biomarkers

Among the oldest and most frequently used biomarkers for predicting a patient's response to antibiotic therapy are fever and leukocytosis. A decline in both indicates that an infectious disease has been adequately treated with a chosen course of antibiotics. More recently, studies have shown that another biomarker, procalcitonin (PCT), can be combined with clinical criteria to help physicians to decide whether to de-escalate or discontinue antibiotic therapy, without affecting outcomes [78]. A systematic review of 26 RCTs involving 6708 participants (acute respiratory infections) from 12 countries found that the duration of antibiotic therapy using PCT concentration reduced mortality, decreased antibiotic consumption, and lowered the risk of antibiotic side-effects. The length of hospital stay and ICU stay were similar in both groups [79]. A randomized trial of 621 patients with suspected community or hospital infection showed that the intervention group (using PCT) had a significantly shorter duration of antibiotic treatment than the control group (14.3 days (SD 9.1) vs. 11.6 days (SD 8.2); absolute difference 2.7 days, 95% CI 1.4 to 4.1, $p < 0.0001$) [80]. Similarly, an RCT of 101 patients with VAP indicated that antibiotic discontinuation based on serum PCT decreased their duration of antibiotic use compared with the control group ($p = 0.038$) [81]. A novel multicenter quality control survey study, including 1759 patients from Switzerland, France, and the United States who had respiratory tract infections, revealed that antibiotic therapy duration based on PCT concentration was shorter than without PCT concentration (5.9 vs. 7.4 days; the absolute difference in days (95% CI), −1.51 (−2.04 to −0.98); $P < 0.001$) [82]. The Infectious Diseases Society of America (IDSA) and the American Thoracic Society (ATS) suggest using PCT levels plus clinical criteria, rather than clinical criteria alone (weak recommendation, low-quality evidence), to guide discontinuation of antibiotic therapy [52].

Besides PCT, another biomarker useful in the management of pneumonia is C-reactive protein (CRP). Together with clinical criteria, low levels of CRP and PCT at 72 h of CAP treatment may improve the prognosis of an absence of severe complications [83]. In a study by Shuren Guo et al., performed on 350 hospitalized CAP patients, CRT and PCT levels on day 3 were statistically lower in the survivors compared to non-survivors [84]. The European Respiratory Society recommended that for patients with suspected pneumonia, along with observing clinical signs and symptoms, a CRP test may be indicated. A CRP level of >100 mg/L, with symptoms for >24 hours makes pneumonia likely; a CRP level < 20 mg/L at presentation, with symptoms for >24 hours, is possibly caused by another respiratory tract infection [85].

Antibiotic resistance is one of the greatest threats to global health, and pneumonia is one of several infections that are becoming less responsive to antibiotic treatment. Antibiotic resistance increases the risk of mortality, prolongs hospital stays, and increases treatment costs. The unnecessary and prolonged use of antibiotics is an important cause contributing to the growth of multidrug-resistant bacteria [86]. This "one size fits all" approach can result in overtreatment, increased side effects, and antibiotic resistance. Therefore, individualization in treatment is important. In addition to clinical assessment, the physician may further consider assessing serum PCT and CRP levels to guide clinical decision-making.

3.3.2 Computerized provider order entry (CPOE) and clinical decision support system (CDSS)

Two useful tools which help in the prevention of ADEs are the computerized physician order entry (CPOE) and clinical decision support systems (CDSS). Compared with conventional medication control, the computerized alert system ADEAS selected different patients based on the risk of an ADE. For the hospital pharmacist, this makes ADEAS a valuable and appropriate tool in reducing the number of preventable ADEs [87].

The implementation of CPOE and advanced CDSS tools substantially increases the number of possible ADE alerts for pharmacist review, and the number of true-positive ADE alerts per 1000 admissions [88].

In a statistical study involving 592 patients during the paper-based prescribing period and 603 patients in the CPOE/CDSS period, the total cost of the paper-based system was €12.37 per patient/day, and of CPOE/CDSS was €14.91 per patient/day. Incremental Cost-Effectiveness Ratios (ICER) for medication errors and for preventable adverse drug events were 3.54 and 322.70, respectively; this indicates the additional amount (€) necessary to prevent a medication error or an ADE. CPOE with primary CDSS contributes to the reduction of the risk of preventable harm. Overall, the additional CPOE/CDSS costs required to prevent medication errors or ADEs appear to be acceptable [89].

However, another study indicated a need to optimize the sensitivity of CPOE/CDSS to detect certain classes of problems, because most DRPs identified by clinical pharmacists were not detected in daily clinical practice by CPOE/CDSS. This underlines the importance of the clinical pharmacist's involvement to reduce DRPs [90].

4. Conclusion

Pneumonia is one of the respiratory diseases causing the highest mortality rate in children and the elderly. As the elderly often have many comorbidities, DRPs also greatly affect their condition and ability to recover.

DRPs in pneumonia are a very complex issue, requiring great attention from healthcare professionals and patients in prescribing, dispensing, and administering medications. Moreover, the rate of hospital readmissions for pneumonia is also a challenging burden, for the health system in general and for patients in particular. The application of technological tools such as CPOE and CDSS to prescribing and ordering can reduce the occurrence of DRPs, but it is physicians, clinical pharmacists and health professionals who play the most important role in reducing DRPs and hospital readmissions in pneumonia.

Author details

Kien T. Nguyen[1], Suol T. Pham[2], Thu P.M. Vo[1*], Chu X. Duong[2],
Dyah A. Perwitasari[3], Ngoc H.K. Truong[4], Dung T.H. Quach[4], Thao N.P. Nguyen[2],
Van T.T. Duong[1], Phuong M. Nguyen[1], Thao H. Nguyen[5], Katja Taxis[6]
and Thang Nguyen[2*]

1 Faculty of Medicine, Can Tho University of Medicine and Pharmacy, Can Tho,
Vietnam

2 Department of Pharmacology and Clinical Pharmacy, Can Tho University of
Medicine and Pharmacy, Can Tho, Vietnam

3 Faculty of Pharmacy, University of Ahmad Dahlan, Yogyakarta, Indonesia

4 College of Natural Sciences, Can Tho University, Can Tho, Vietnam

5 Department of Clinical Pharmacy, University of Medicine and Pharmacy at Ho
Chi Minh City, Ho Chi Minh City, Vietnam

6 Groningen Research Institute of Pharmacy, University of Groningen, Groningen,
The Netherlands

*Address all correspondence to: vpmthu@ctump.edu.vn and nthang@ctump.edu.vn

IntechOpen

References

[1] Pneumonia [Internet]. Available from: https://www.who.int/westernpacific/health-topics/pneumonia [Accessed: 2021-07-17]

[2] Pneumonia in Children Statistics [Internet]. UNICEF DATA. Available from: https://data.unicef.org/topic/child-health/pneumonia/[Accessed: 2021-07-17]

[3] Jain S, Self WH, Wunderink RG, Fakhran S, Balk R, Bramley AM, et al. Community-Acquired Pneumonia Requiring Hospitalization among U.S. Adults. N Engl J Med. 2015 Jul 30;373(5):415-27. DOI: 10.1056/NEJMoa1500245

[4] Takahashi K, Suzuki M, Minh LN, Anh NH, Huong LTM, Son TVV, et al. The incidence and aetiology of hospitalised community-acquired pneumonia among Vietnamese adults: a prospective surveillance in Central Vietnam. BMC Infectious Diseases. 2013 Jul 1;13(1):296. DOI: 10.1186/1471-2334-13-296

[5] Azmi S, Aljunid SM, Maimaiti N, Ali A-A, Muhammad Nur A, De Rosas-Valera M, et al. Assessing the burden of pneumonia using administrative data from Malaysia, Indonesia, and the Philippines. International Journal of Infectious Diseases. 2016 Aug 1;49:87-93. DOI: 10.1016/j.ijid.2016.05.021

[6] Working groups items - Pharmaceutical Care Network Europe [Internet]. Available from: https://www.pcne.org/working-groups/2/drug-related-problems [Accessed: 2021-07-17]

[7] 417_PCNE_classification_V9-1_final.pdf [Internet]. Available from: https://www.pcne.org/upload/files/417_PCNE_classification_V9-1_final.pdf [Accessed: 2021-07-17]

[8] Kuti EL, Patel AA, Coleman CI. Impact of inappropriate antibiotic therapy on mortality in patients with ventilator-associated pneumonia and blood stream infection: A meta-analysis. Journal of Critical Care. 2008 Mar 1;23(1):91-100. DOI: 10.1016/j.jcrc.2007.08.007

[9] Guillamet CV, Vazquez R, Noe J, Micek ST, Kollef MH. A cohort study of bacteremic pneumonia: The importance of antibiotic resistance and appropriate initial therapy? Medicine. 2016 Aug;95(35):e4708. DOI: 10.1097/MD.0000000000004708

[10] Bekele F, Fekadu G, Bekele K, Dugassa D, Sori J. Drug-related problems among patients with infectious disease admitted to medical wards of Wollega University Referral Hospital: Prospective observational study. SAGE Open Med. 2021;9:2050312121989625. DOI: 10.1177/2050312121989625

[11] Garin N, Sole N, Lucas B, Matas L, Moras D, Rodrigo-Troyano A, et al. Drug related problems in clinical practice: a cross-sectional study on their prevalence, risk factors and associated pharmaceutical interventions. Sci Rep. 2021 Jan 13;11(1):883. DOI: 10.1038/s41598-020-80560-2

[12] Ngocho JS, Horumpende PG, de Jonge MI, Mmbaga BT. Inappropriate treatment of community-acquired pneumonia among children under five years of age in Tanzania. Int J Infect Dis. 2020 Apr;93:56-61. DOI: 10.1016/j.ijid.2020.01.038

[13] Roberts JA, Paul SK, Akova M, Bassetti M, De Waele JJ, Dimopoulos G, et al. DALI: defining antibiotic levels in intensive care unit patients: are current β-lactam antibiotic doses sufficient for critically ill patients? Clin Infect Dis. 2014 Apr;58(8):1072-83. DOI: 10.1093/cid/ciu027

[14] Daneman N, Gruneir A, Bronskill SE, Newman A, Fischer HD, Rochon PA, et al. Prolonged Antibiotic Treatment in Long-term Care: Role of the Prescriber. JAMA Intern Med. 2013 Apr 22;173(8):673. DOI: 10.1001/jamainternmed.2013.3029

[15] Noor S, Ismail M, Ali Z. Potential drug-drug interactions among pneumonia patients: do these matter in clinical perspectives? BMC Pharmacology and Toxicology. 2019 Jul 26;20(1):45. DOI: 10.1186/s40360-019-0325-7

[16] Wunderink RG, Srinivasan A, Barie PS, Chastre J, Dela Cruz CS, Douglas IS, et al. Antibiotic Stewardship in the Intensive Care Unit. An Official American Thoracic Society Workshop Report in Collaboration with the AACN, CHEST, CDC, and SCCM. Annals ATS. 2020 May;17(5):531-40. DOI: 10.1513/AnnalsATS.202003-188ST

[17] Oliver MB, Fong K, Certain L, Spivak ES, Timbrook TT. Validation of a Community-Acquired Pneumonia Score To Improve Empiric Antibiotic Selection at an Academic Medical Center. Antimicrob Agents Chemother. 2021 Jan 20;65(2):e01482-20. DOI: 10.1128/AAC.01482-20

[18] Bell BG, Schellevis F, Stobberingh E, Goossens H, Pringle M. A systematic review and meta-analysis of the effects of antibiotic consumption on antibiotic resistance. BMC Infect Dis. 2014 Jan 9;14:13. DOI: 10.1186/1471-2334-14-13

[19] Cara AKS, Zaidi STR, Suleman F. Cost-effectiveness analysis of low versus high dose colistin in the treatment of multi-drug resistant pneumonia in Saudi Arabia. Int J Clin Pharm. 2018 Oct;40(5):1051-8. DOI: 10.1007/s11096-018-0713-x

[20] Dorj G, Hendrie D, Parsons R, Sunderland B. An evaluation of prescribing practices for

community-acquired pneumonia (CAP) in Mongolia. BMC Health Serv Res. 2013 Oct 3;13(1):379. DOI: 10.1186/1472-6963-13-379

[21] Wattengel BA, Sellick JA, Skelly MK, Napierala R, Schroeck J, Mergenhagen KA. Outpatient Antimicrobial Stewardship: Targets for Community-acquired Pneumonia. Clinical Therapeutics. 2019 Mar;41(3):466-76. DOI: 10.1016/j.clinthera.2019.01.007

[22] Wongsurakiat P, Chitwarakorn N. Severe community-acquired pneumonia in general medical wards: outcomes and impact of initial antibiotic selection. BMC Pulm Med. 2019 Dec;19(1):179. DOI: 10.1186/s12890-019-0944-1

[23] Leone M, Garcin F, Bouvenot J, Boyadjev I, Visintini P, Albanèse J, et al. Ventilator-associated pneumonia: breaking the vicious circle of antibiotic overuse. Crit Care Med. 2007 Feb;35(2):379-85; quizz 386. DOI: 10.1097/01.CCM.0000253404.69418.AA

[24] Postma DF, van Werkhoven CH, van Elden LJR, Thijsen SFT, Hoepelman AIM, Kluytmans JAJW, et al. Antibiotic Treatment Strategies for Community-Acquired Pneumonia in Adults. New England Journal of Medicine. 2015 Apr 2;372(14):1312-23. DOI: 10.1056/NEJMoa1406330

[25] Tumbarello M, Trecarichi EM, Tumietto F, Del Bono V, De Rosa FG, Bassetti M, et al. Predictive models for identification of hospitalized patients harboring KPC-producing *Klebsiella pneumoniae*. Antimicrob Agents Chemother. 2014 Jun;58(6):3514-20. DOI: 10.1128/AAC.02373-13

[26] Bradley JS, Byington CL, Shah SS, Alverson B, Carter ER, Harrison C, et al. The Management of Community-Acquired Pneumonia in Infants and Children Older Than 3 Months of Age: Clinical Practice Guidelines by the

Pediatric Infectious Diseases Society and the Infectious Diseases Society of America. Clinical Infectious Diseases. 2011 Oct 1;53(7):e25-76. DOI: 10.1093/cid/cir531

[27] Gralnek I, Dumonceau J-M, Kuipers E, Lanas A, Sanders D, Kurien M, et al. Diagnosis and management of nonvariceal upper gastrointestinal hemorrhage: European Society of Gastrointestinal Endoscopy (ESGE) Guideline. Endoscopy. 2015 Sep 29;47(10):a1-46. DOI: 10.1055/s-0034-1393172

[28] Thiessen K, Lloyd AE, Miller MJ, Homco J, Gildon B, O'Neal KS. Assessing guideline-concordant prescribing for community-acquired pneumonia. Int J Clin Pharm. 2017 Aug;39(4):674-8. DOI: 10.1007/s11096-017-0489-4

[29] Yu J, Wang G, Davidson A, Chow I, Chiu A. Antibiotics Utilization for Community Acquired Pneumonia in a Community Hospital Emergency Department. Journal of Pharmacy Practice. 2020 Sep 10;089719002095303. DOI: 10.1177/0897190020953032

[30] Research C for DE and. FDA reinforces safety information about serious low blood sugar levels and mental health side effects with fluoroquinolone antibiotics; requires label changes. FDA [Internet]. 2019 Apr 15. Available from: https://www.fda.gov/drugs/drug-safety-and-availability/fda-reinforces-safety-information-about-serious-low-blood-sugar-levels-and-mental-health-side [Accessed: 2021-06-21]

[31] Research C for DE and. FDA warns about increased risk of ruptures or tears in the aorta blood vessel with fluoroquinolone antibiotics in certain patients. FDA [Internet]. 2019 Dec 20. Available from: https://www.fda.gov/drugs/drug-safety-and-availability/fda-warns-about-increased-risk-ruptures-or-tears-aorta-blood-vessel-fluoroquinolone-antibiotics [Accessed: 2021-06-23]

[32] Torumkuney D, Van PH, Thinh LQ, Koo SH, Tan SH, Lim PQ, et al. Results from the Survey of Antibiotic Resistance (SOAR) 2016-18 in Vietnam, Cambodia, Singapore and the Philippines: data based on CLSI, EUCAST (dose-specific) and pharmacokinetic/pharmacodynamic (PK/PD) breakpoints. Journal of Antimicrobial Chemotherapy. 2020 Apr 1;75(Supplement_1):i19-42. DOI: 10.1093/jac/dkaa082

[33] Kulwicki BD, Brandt KL, Wolf LM, Weise AJ, Dumkow LE. Impact of an emergency medicine pharmacist on empiric antibiotic prescribing for pneumonia and intra-abdominal infections. The American Journal of Emergency Medicine. 2019 May;37(5):839-44. DOI: 10.1016/j.ajem.2018.07.052

[34] Galanter KM, Ho J. Impact of an empiric therapy guide on antibiotic prescribing in the emergency department. Journal of Hospital Infection. 2020 Feb;104(2):188-92. DOI: 10.1016/j.jhin.2019.09.017

[35] Gamble J-M, Hall JJ, Marrie TJ, Sadowski CA, Majumdar SR, Eurich DT. Medication transitions and polypharmacy in older adults following acute care. TCRM. 2014 Mar 19;10:189-96. DOI: 10.2147/TCRM.S58707

[36] Wesemann T, Nüllmann H, Pflug MA, Heppner HJ, Pientka L, Thiem U. Pneumonia severity, comorbidity and 1-year mortality in predominantly older adults with community-acquired pneumonia: a cohort study. BMC Infectious Diseases. 2015 Jan 8;15(1):2. DOI: 10.1186/s12879-014-0730-x

[37] Henig O, Kaye KS. Bacterial Pneumonia in Older Adults. Infectious

Disease Clinics of North America. 2017 Dec 1;31(4):689-713. DOI: 10.1016/j.idc.2017.07.015

[38] Gülçebi İdriz Oğlu M, Küçükibrahimoğlu E, Karaalp A, Sarikaya Ö, Demirkapu M, Onat F, et al. Potential drug-drug interactions in a medical intensive care unit of a university hospital. Turk J Med Sci. 2016 Apr 19;46(3):812-9. DOI: 10.3906/sag-1504-147

[39] Lodise TP, Zhao Q, Fahrbach K, Gillard PJ, Martin A. A systematic review of the association between delayed appropriate therapy and mortality among patients hospitalized with infections due to *Klebsiella pneumoniae* or *Escherichia coli*: how long is too long? BMC Infect Dis. 2018 Dec;18(1):625. DOI: 10.1186/s12879-018-3524-8

[40] Iregui M, Ward S, Sherman G, Fraser VJ, Kollef MH. Clinical Importance of Delays in the Initiation of Appropriate Antibiotic Treatment for Ventilator-Associated Pneumonia. Chest. 2002 Jul;122(1):262-8. DOI: 10.1378/chest.122.1.262

[41] Lim WS, Baudouin SV, George RC, Hill AT, Jamieson C, Jeune IL, et al. BTS guidelines for the management of community acquired pneumonia in adults: update 2009. Thorax. 2009 Oct 1;64(Suppl 3):iii1-55. DOI: 10.1136/thx.2009.121434

[42] Daniel P, Rodrigo C, Mckeever TM, Woodhead M, Welham S, Lim WS. Time to first antibiotic and mortality in adults hospitalised with community-acquired pneumonia: a matched-propensity analysis. Thorax. 2016 Jun 1;71(6):568-70. DOI: 10.1136/thoraxjnl-2015-207513

[43] Houck PM, Bratzler DW, Nsa W, Ma A, Bartlett JG. Timing of Antibiotic Administration and Outcomes for Medicare Patients Hospitalized With Community-Acquired Pneumonia. Arch Intern Med. 2004 Mar 22;164(6):637. DOI: 10.1001/archinte.164.6.637

[44] Spellberg B. The New Antibiotic Mantra—"Shorter Is Better." JAMA Intern Med. 2016 Sep 1;176(9):1254-5. DOI: 10.1001/jamainternmed.2016.3646

[45] Metlay JP, Waterer GW, Long AC, Anzueto A, Brozek J, Crothers K, et al. Diagnosis and Treatment of Adults with Community-acquired Pneumonia. An Official Clinical Practice Guideline of the American Thoracic Society and Infectious Diseases Society of America. Am J Respir Crit Care Med. 2019 Oct 1;200(7):e45-67. DOI: 10.1164/rccm.201908-1581ST

[46] Gaynes R, Rimland D, Killum E, Lowery HK, Johnson TM, Killgore G, et al. Outbreak of *Clostridium difficile* infection in a long-term care facility: association with gatifloxacin use. Clin Infect Dis. 2004 Mar 1;38(5):640-5. DOI: 10.1086/381551

[47] Chastre J, Wolff M, Fagon J-Y, Chevret S, Thomas F, Wermert D, et al. Comparison of 8 vs 15 Days of Antibiotic Therapy for Ventilator-Associated Pneumonia in Adults: A Randomized Trial. JAMA. 2003 Nov 19;290(19):2588. DOI: 10.1001/jama.290.19.2588

[48] Yi SH, Hatfield KM, Baggs J, Hicks LA, Srinivasan A, Reddy S, et al. Duration of Antibiotic Use Among Adults With Uncomplicated Community-Acquired Pneumonia Requiring Hospitalization in the United States. Clinical Infectious Diseases. 2018 Apr 17;66(9):1333-41. DOI: 10.1093/cid/cix986

[49] Madaras-Kelly KJ, Burk M, Caplinger C, Bohan JG, Neuhauser MM, Goetz MB, et al. Total duration of antimicrobial therapy in veterans hospitalized with uncomplicated pneumonia: Results of a national medication utilization evaluation:

Pneumonia Treatment Duration. J Hosp Med. 2016 Dec;11(12):832-9. DOI: 10.1002/jhm.2648

[50] Pugh R, Grant C, Cooke RPD, Dempsey G. Short-course versus prolonged-course antibiotic therapy for hospital-acquired pneumonia in critically ill adults. Cochrane Database Syst Rev. 2015 Aug 24;(8):CD007577. DOI: 10.1002/14651858.CD007577.pub3

[51] Mathur NB, Murugesan A. Comparison of Four Days Versus Seven Days Duration of Antibiotic Therapy for Neonatal Pneumonia: A Randomized Controlled Trial. Indian J Pediatr. 2018 Nov;85(11):963-7. DOI: 10.1007/s12098-018-2708-y

[52] Kalil AC, Metersky ML, Klompas M, Muscedere J, Sweeney DA, Palmer LB, et al. Management of Adults With Hospital-acquired and Ventilator-associated Pneumonia: 2016 Clinical Practice Guidelines by the Infectious Diseases Society of America and the American Thoracic Society. Clinical Infectious Diseases. 2016 Sep 1;63(5):e61-111. DOI: 10.1093/cid/ciw353

[53] Karakioulaki M, Stolz D. Biomarkers and clinical scoring systems in community-acquired pneumonia. Ann Thorac Med. 2019;14(3):165. DOI: 10.4103/atm.ATM_305_18

[54] Foolad F, Huang AM, Nguyen CT, Colyer L, Lim M, Grieger J, et al. A multicentre stewardship initiative to decrease excessive duration of antibiotic therapy for the treatment of community-acquired pneumonia. Journal of Antimicrobial Chemotherapy. 2018 May 1;73(5):1402-7. DOI: 10.1093/jac/dky021

[55] Menditto E, Gimeno Miguel A, Moreno Juste A, Poblador Plou B, Aza Pascual-Salcedo M, Orlando V, et al. Patterns of multimorbidity and polypharmacy in young and adult population: Systematic associations among chronic diseases and drugs using factor analysis. PLoS One. 2019;14(2):e0210701. DOI: 10.1371/journal.pone.0210701

[56] Yousufuddin M, Shultz J, Doyle T, Rehman H, Murad MH. Incremental risk of long-term mortality with increased burden of comorbidity in hospitalized patients with pneumonia. European Journal of Internal Medicine. 2018 Sep 1;55:23-7. DOI: 10.1016/j.ejim.2018.05.003

[57] Hespanhol V, Bárbara C. Pneumonia mortality, comorbidities matter? Pulmonology. 2020 Jun;26(3):123-9. DOI: [51]

[58] Franzen D, Lim M, Bratton DJ, Kuster SP, Kohler M. The Roles of the Charlson Comorbidity Index and Time to First Antibiotic Dose as Predictors of Outcome in Pneumococcal Community-Acquired Pneumonia. Lung. 2016 Oct;194(5):769-75. DOI: 10.1007/s00408-016-9922-z

[59] Nguyen MTN, Saito N, Wagatsuma Y. The effect of comorbidities for the prognosis of community-acquired pneumonia: an epidemiologic study using a hospital surveillance in Japan. BMC Res Notes. 2019 Dec 19;12(1):817. DOI: 10.1186/s13104-019-4848-1

[60] Aurilio RB, Sant'Anna CC, March M de FBP. CLINICAL PROFILE OF CHILDREN WITH AND WITHOUT COMORBIDITIES HOSPITALIZED WITH COMMUNITY-ACQUIRED PNEUMONIA. Rev Paul Pediatr. 2020;38:e2018333. DOI: 10.1590/1984-0462/2020/38/2018333

[61] El Morabet N, Uitvlugt EB, van den Bemt BJF, van den Bemt PMLA, Janssen MJA, Karapinar-Çarkit F. Prevalence and Preventability of Drug-Related Hospital Readmissions:

A Systematic Review. J Am Geriatr Soc. 2018 Mar;66(3):602-8. DOI: 10.1111/jgs.15244

[62] Saldanha V, Araújo IB de, Lima SIVC, Martins RR, Oliveira AG. Risk factors for drug-related problems in a general hospital: A large prospective cohort. PLoS One. 2020;15(5):e0230215. DOI: 10.1371/journal.pone.0230215

[63] Abou-Karam N, Bradford C, Lor KB, Barnett M, Ha M, Rizos A. Medication regimen complexity and readmissions after hospitalization for heart failure, acute myocardial infarction, pneumonia, and chronic obstructive pulmonary disease. SAGE Open Med. 2016;4:2050312116632426. DOI: [37]

[64] Willson MN, Greer CL, Weeks DL. Medication regimen complexity and hospital readmission for an adverse drug event. Ann Pharmacother. 2014 Jan;48(1):26-32. DOI: 10.1177/1060028013510898

[65] Jang JG, Ahn JH. Reasons and Risk Factors for Readmission Following Hospitalization for Community-acquired Pneumonia in South Korea. Tuberc Respir Dis (Seoul). 2020 Apr;83(2):147-56. DOI: 10.4046/trd.2019.0073

[66] Faverio P, Compagnoni MM, Della Zoppa M, Pesci A, Cantarutti A, Merlino L, et al. Rehospitalization for pneumonia after first pneumonia admission: Incidence and predictors in a population-based cohort study. PLoS One. 2020;15(6):e0235468. DOI: 10.1371/journal.pone.0235468

[67] Wang L, Feng Z, Shuai J, Liu J, Li G. Risk factors of 90-day rehospitalization following discharge of pediatric patients hospitalized with *mycoplasma Pneumoniae* pneumonia. BMC Infectious Diseases. 2019 Nov 12;19(1):966. DOI: 10.1186/s12879-019-4616-9

[68] Toledo D, Soldevila N, Torner N, Pérez-Lozano MJ, Espejo E, Navarro G, et al. Factors associated with 30-day readmission after hospitalisation for community-acquired pneumonia in older patients: a cross-sectional study in seven Spanish regions. BMJ Open. 2018 Mar 30;8(3):e020243. DOI: 10.1136/bmjopen-2017-020243

[69] Lisenby KM, Carroll DN, Pinner NA. Evaluation of a Pharmacist-Specific Intervention on 30-Day Readmission Rates for High-Risk Patients with Pneumonia. Hosp Pharm. 2015 Sep;50(8):700-9. DOI: 10.1310/hpj5008-700

[70] Gil R, Webb BJ. Strategies for prediction of drug-resistant pathogens and empiric antibiotic selection in community-acquired pneumonia. Curr Opin Pulm Med. 2020 May;26(3):249-59. DOI: 10.1097/MCP.0000000000000670

[71] McGowan JJ, Gerding DN. Does antibiotic restriction prevent resistance. New Horiz. 1996 Aug 1;4(3):370-6. PMID: 8856755

[72] Fishman N, America S for HE of, America IDS of, Society PID. Policy Statement on Antimicrobial Stewardship by the Society for Healthcare Epidemiology of America (SHEA), the Infectious Diseases Society of America (IDSA), and the Pediatric Infectious Diseases Society (PIDS). Infection Control & Hospital Epidemiology. 2012 Apr;33(4):322-7. DOI: 10.1086/665010

[73] Uranga A, España PP, Bilbao A, Quintana JM, Arriaga I, Intxausti M, et al. Duration of Antibiotic Treatment in Community-Acquired Pneumonia: A Multicenter Randomized Clinical Trial. JAMA Intern Med. 2016 Sep 1;176(9):1257-65. DOI: 10.1001/jamainternmed.2016.3633

[74] CDC. The Core Elements of Hospital Antibiotic Stewardship

Programs. Atlanta, GA: US Department of Health and Human Services [Internet]. CDC; 2019. Available from: https://www.cdc.gov/antibiotic-use/core-elements/hospital.html. [Accessed: 2021-08-05]

[75] EML_2017_ExecutiveSummary.pdf [Internet]. Available from: https://www.who.int/medicines/publications/essentialmedicines/EML_2017_ExecutiveSummary.pdf [Accessed: 2021-08-07]

[76] Chung GW, Wu JE, Yeo CL, Chan D, Hsu LY. Antimicrobial stewardship: a review of prospective audit and feedback systems and an objective evaluation of outcomes. Virulence. 2013 Feb 15;4(2):151-7. DOI: 10.4161/viru.21626

[77] VanLangen KM, Dumkow LE, Axford KL, Havlichek DH, Baker JJ, Drobish IC, et al. Evaluation of a multifaceted approach to antimicrobial stewardship education methods for medical residents. Infect Control Hosp Epidemiol. 2019 Nov;40(11):1236-41. DOI: 10.1017/ice.2019.253

[78] Bennett JE, Dolin R, Blaser MJ, editors. Mandell, Douglas, and Bennett's principles and practice of infectious diseases. Ninth edition. Philadelphia, PA: Elsevier; 2020. 216p. ISBN: 978-0-323-48255-4

[79] Schuetz P, Wirz Y, Sager R, Christ-Crain M, Stolz D, Tamm M, et al. Procalcitonin to initiate or discontinue antibiotics in acute respiratory tract infections. Cochrane Database Syst Rev. 2017 Oct 12;10:CD007498. DOI: 10.1002/14651858.CD007498.pub3

[80] Bouadma L, Luyt C-E, Tubach F, Cracco C, Alvarez A, Schwebel C, et al. Use of procalcitonin to reduce patients' exposure to antibiotics in intensive care units (PRORATA trial): a multicentre randomised controlled trial. The Lancet. 2010 Feb 6;375(9713):463-74. DOI: 10.1016/S0140-6736(09)61879-1

[81] Stolz D, Smyrnios N, Eggimann P, Pargger H, Thakkar N, Siegemund M, et al. Procalcitonin for reduced antibiotic exposure in ventilator-associated pneumonia: a randomised study. European Respiratory Journal. 2009 Dec 1;34(6):1364-75. DOI: 10.1183/09031936.00053209

[82] Albrich WC, Dusemund F, Bucher B, Meyer S, Thomann R, Kühn F, et al. Effectiveness and safety of procalcitonin-guided antibiotic therapy in lower respiratory tract infections in "real life": an international, multicenter poststudy survey (ProREAL). Arch Intern Med. 2012 May 14;172(9):715-22. DOI: 10.1001/archinternmed.2012.770

[83] Menéndez R, Martinez R, Reyes S, Mensa J, Polverino E, Filella X, et al. Stability in community-acquired pneumonia: one step forward with markers? Thorax. 2009 Nov;64(11):987-92. DOI: [65]

[84] Guo S, Mao X, Liang M. The moderate predictive value of serial serum CRP and PCT levels for the prognosis of hospitalized community-acquired pneumonia. Respiratory Research. 2018 Oct 1;19(1):193. DOI: 10.1186/s12931-018-0877-x

[85] Woodhead M, Blasi F, Ewig S, Garau J, Huchon G, Ieven M, et al. Guidelines for the management of adult lower respiratory tract infections - Full version. Clin Microbiol Infect. 2011 Nov;17(Suppl 6):E1-59. DOI: 10.1111/j.1469-0691.2011.03672.x

[86] Antibiotic resistance [Internet]. Available from: https://www.who.int/news-room/fact-sheets/detail/antibiotic-resistance [Accessed: 2021-07-14]

[87] Rommers MK, Teepe-Twiss IM, Guchelaar H-J. A computerized adverse drug event alerting system using clinical rules: a retrospective and prospective comparison with conventional

medication surveillance in the
Netherlands. Drug Saf. 2011 Mar
1;34(3):233-42. DOI:
10.2165/11536500-000000000-00000

[88] Roberts LL, Ward MM, Brokel JM,
Wakefield DS, Crandall DK, Conlon P.
Impact of health information
technology on detection of potential
adverse drug events at the ordering
stage. Am J Health Syst Pharm. 2010
Nov 1;67(21):1838-46. DOI: 10.2146/
ajhp090637

[89] Vermeulen KM, van Doormaal JE,
Zaal RJ, Mol PGM, Lenderink AW,
Haaijer-Ruskamp FM, et al. Cost-
effectiveness of an electronic
medication ordering system (CPOE/
CDSS) in hospitalized patients. Int J
Med Inform. 2014 Aug;83(8):572-80.
DOI: 10.1016/j.ijmedinf.2014.05.003

[90] Zaal RJ, Jansen MMPM,
Duisenberg-van Essenberg M,
Tijssen CC, Roukema JA, van den
Bemt PMLA. Identification of drug-
related problems by a clinical
pharmacist in addition to computerized
alerts. Int J Clin Pharm. 2013
Oct;35(5):753-62. DOI: 10.1007/
s11096-013-9798-4

Chapter 4

Examining the Executioners, Influenza Associated Secondary Bacterial Pneumonia

Timothy R. Borgogna and Jovanka M. Voyich

Abstract

Influenza infections typically present mild to moderate morbidities in immunocompetent host and are often resolved within 14 days of infection onset. Death from influenza infection alone is uncommon; however, antecedent influenza infection often leads to an increased susceptibility to secondary bacterial pneumonia. Bacterial pneumonia following viral infection exhibits mortality rates greater than 10-fold of those of influenza alone. Furthermore, bacterial pneumonia has been identified as the major contributor to mortality during each of the previous four influenza pandemics. *Streptococcus pneumoniae*, *Staphylococcus aureus*, *Haemophilus influenzae*, and *Streptococcus pyogenes* are the most prevalent participants in this pathology. Of note, these lung pathogens are frequently found as commensals of the upper respiratory tract. Herein we describe influenza-induced host-changes that lead to increased susceptibility to bacterial pneumonia, review virulence strategies employed by the most prevalent secondary bacterial pneumonia species, and highlight recent findings of bacterial sensing and responding to the influenza infected environment.

Keywords: pneumonia, influenza, *Streptococcus pneumoniae*, *Staphylococcus aureus*, *Haemophilus influenzae*, *Streptococcus pyogenes*, co-infection, superinfection, secondary pneumonia

1. Introduction

It starts mild. Congestion, fever, body aches, and fatigue. Influenza is infecting the respiratory tract. Seven days and relief should be on the horizon, but the days pass and the symptoms worsen. Breathing becomes laborious and the insides burn with a fire. Crackling can be heard as the stethoscope is pressed against the chest. The sequence of events to follow is all too common. Soon the lungs will be too weak to fulfill their function. The infection will disseminate, shutting down the organs in its path. Multisystem organ failure ensues and secondary bacterial pneumonia adds another mark to its resumé.

Unlike many diseases that have plagued human past, influenza continues to remain a prominent threat and leading cause of worldwide morbidity and mortality. The etiology of influenza would be task for the 20th century, but descriptions of influenza-like diseases and pandemics begin as early as ca 410 BCE [1, 2]. Accurate reports of disease are scarce through early middle-ages, however, descriptions of an epidemic spreading through Britain in CE 664 have been attributed to influenza [3]. England, France, and Italy are thought to have experienced an influenza pandemic from 1173 to 1174. Contemporaries of this period reported "...an inflammatory plague spread... and all eyes swept following a cruel rhinorrhea" [3, 4]. A community in Florence, Italy in 1357 associated a seasonality to the abrupt onset of symptoms—fatigue, fever, and catarrh—with the changing weather of the winter months; collectively members of community termed the disease "*influenza di freddo*" or "influence from cold," giving rise to the diagnostic term, "influenza" [3, 5].

Around 1500, descriptions of influenza become more consistent. Notably, it is now accepted that during his second journey to the new world in 1493, Christopher Columbus and his crew were suffering from influenza. Upon reaching the Antilles, influenza spread from the crew to the native population killing an estimated 90% of indigenous inhabitants [6, 7]. This was the first report of influenza spreading from Europe across the Atlantic Ocean, a trait that would soon become a hallmark of its infectivity. Reports of epidemics arising throughout Europe and spreading into the Americas were observed in 1658, 1679, 1708, and 1729 and would continue into the 1800s; however, it was the devastating impact of the influenza pandemic of 1918 that would forever influence modern research and understanding on influenza associated pneumonia [3, 8].

The 1918 influenza pandemic has been referred to as "the greatest medical holocaust in history" [2]. Conservative estimates report the 1918 influenza strain led to 50 million global deaths while others suggest the death toll could have reached as many as 100 million [9]. At the time of the 1918 outbreak, the etiological agent of influenza had yet to be correctly identified. Despite this, contemporary physicians had observed that the increases in influenza mortalities were not due to influenza alone. In a letter to a colleague, Dr. Roy Grist states, "There is no doubt in my mind that there is a new mixed infection here, but what I do not know" [10]. Similarly, in reference to increases in influenza-associated deaths, Louis Cruveilheir made the infamous confession, "If grippe condemns, the secondary infections execute" [11].

In the previous decades Richard Pfeiffer had isolated a rod-shaped bacterium from the nose of flu-infected patients that he believed to be the causative agent of influenza [12]. Pfieffer named the bacterium *Bacillus influenzae* which would later come to be known as *H. influenzae* [12]. Though Pfieffer's work was widely accepted, the devastation accompanying the 1918 pandemic caused renewed vigor in influenza research that ultimately called into question the validity of Pfieffer's claims. In 1921 Peter Olitsky and Fredericck Gates took nasal secretions from patients infected from the 1918 strain and passed them through a Berkefeld filter. The filtrate, presumably devoid of bacteria, was then exposed to rabbits wherein the rabbits subsequently demonstrated symptoms indicative of an influenza infection [12, 13]. Olitsky and Gates' studies were the first to suggest the causative agent of influenza was not of bacterial origin, but their work became heavily criticized as others struggled to repeat it. It wasn't until 1929 that Richard Shope, following Olitsky and Gates' filtration method, would use lung samples from an influenza infected pig to demonstrate that the filterable agent was the cause of the influenza, thus ending the debate on bacterial influenza [12, 14]. In the same journal issue that Shope published his findings regarding the causative agent of influenza, he published a separate article describing that swine infected with influenza displayed an increased susceptibility to bacterial infection [15]. While the significance of this finding would not be fully realized for nearly 100 years, Shope had identified the leading cause of influenza associated mortalities—secondary bacterial pneumonia.

2. Influenza pandemics and secondary bacterial pneumonia

Influenza is a prominent global pathogen responsible for an estimated 1 billion infections annually [16–18]. Despite maintaining high infection rates, mortalities due to influenza infection alone are infrequent. In most immunocompetent hosts, infections cause mild to moderate morbidities and are often resolved within 14-days of symptom onset; however, infection with influenza markedly increases host susceptibility to secondary bacterial infection [11, 19–22]. Cases such as these often display mortality rates between 10 and 15-fold greater than those of influenza alone [23–26].

Modern studies examining the samples from the four most recent influenza pandemics (1918, 1957, 1968, and 2009) demonstrated up to 95% of fatal cases were associated with secondary bacterial infections [11, 22, 27]. The dominant causative agents of this pathology have been *S. aureus* (*S. aureus*), *S. pneumoniae* (*S. pneumoniae*), and to a lesser extent *H. influenzae* (*H. influenzae*) [11, 22, 28]. Each of the previous pandemics demonstrated a unique predisposition for secondary bacterial infection with specific species. For example, bacterial pneumonia associated with the 1918 H1N1 pandemic was dominated by *S. pneumoniae*; conversely the 1957, H2N2 pandemic was dominated by *S. aureus* [28]. Both *S. pneumoniae* and *S. aureus* were highly prominent in the 1968 H3N2 related bacterial infections, however, infections with *S. pneumoniae* were slightly more common. In the most recent 2009 H1N1 outbreak cases associated with *S. pneumoniae* and *S. aureus* were nearly equivalent [28].

Comparative genetic analysis of seasonal and pandemic influenza viruses has highlighted the importance of the PB1-F2 protein in increased inflammation and susceptibility to secondary bacterial pneumonia; however, the mechanisms defining the associations between different strains of influenza and specific bacterial pathogens remain incompletely defined [29–31]. Differences between bacterial agents following antecedent influenza infection were first described in the immediate wake of the 1957 pandemic. Two distinct pathologies of bacterial infection were observed. In the first, bacterial infection arose after viral clearance and were highly dominated by *S. pneumoniae*. In the second, bacterial infection occurred during the viral infection and were predominantly caused by *S. aureus*. Patients inflicted with superinfections by *S. aureus* represented the majority of severe and fatal cases [32]. Of note, this pattern of infection sequence and outcome is consistent with current observations. It is now generally recognized that *S. pneumoniae* is the most prevalent cause of secondary bacterial infection whereas *S. aureus* has emerged as the most common cause of severe and life-threatening cases [22, 27, 33, 34].

2.1 Dysregulation of innate immunity

The prevalent etiological agents of bacterial pneumonia following antecedent influenza infection (*S. aureus*, *S. pneumoniae*, and *H. influenzae*) are common, persistent, and asymptomatic colonizers of upper respiratory tract [35–38]. Curiously, this is a trait shared by other microorganisms that are less frequent causes of secondary pneumonia such as *S. pyogenes* (*S. pyogenes*) [38, 39]. Studies examining the contributions of respiratory commensals on lower respiratory disease have revealed residents of the upper respiratory tract are frequently trafficked into the lungs via inhalation, microaspirations, and direct mucosal dispersion [40, 41]. Despite recurrent exposure to the lower respiratory environment, and apart from a preceding influenza infection, bacterial pneumonia in immune competent adults is uncommon [21, 22, 42]. This has prompted many studies aimed at understanding influenza induced dysregulations in immune function that lead to increases in susceptibility to bacterial infection. To that end, considerable progress has been made identifying key changes within the host environment that prelude bacterial pneumonia [21, 43, 44].

In general, susceptibility to bacterial co-infection peaks 6–7 days post influenza infection and corresponds with increases in tissue damage and dysregulation of cytokine production [36, 45, 46]. In immunocompetent individuals, alveolar macrophages and neutrophils are the primary cell types responsible for controlling bacteria invading the lower respiratory tract (LRT). During influenza infection the bactericidal activity of these two cells is severely impaired [47–50]. Specifically, influenza infection can cause a ≥85% loss in alveolar macrophages numbers by day 7 of the infection [47, 51]. Aberrant interferon-gamma (IFN-γ) signaling in the macrophages that are present demonstrate impaired phagocytic activity [48]. Similarly, the incumbent infection elicits production of the regulatory cytokine IL-10 in the lung epithelia. IL-10 reduces phagocytic activity in neutrophils [36, 43, 52]. Pretreatment of mice with a neutralizing monoclonal antibody against IL-10 after viral infection, but prior to onset of bacterial infection, significantly increases mouse survival [34]. Other notable immunological changes implicated in increased susceptibility to secondary bacterial infection include disruptions in the TH17 pathway, type-I IFN production, and antimicrobial peptide production [53–59]. While these studies certainly contribute to identifying factors leading to the increased susceptibility to secondary bacterial pneumonia following influenza infection, they fail to address the direct impacts of the viral infection on the pathogenesis of these bacterial species.

2.2 Viral influence on bacterial virulence

Given the frequency of upper respiratory colonization with bacterial pathobionts and the opportunity for exposure into the lower respiratory environment, it is shocking that severe bacteria pneumonia is not more common. Moreover, it is often overlooked that these species contain a diverse repertoire of virulence factors that must be suppressed during colonization to avoid a host response. Recent models of infection have enabled investigators to begin to examine how influenza infections can promote transcriptional changes leading to a transition from asymptomatic commensal to life-threatening pathogen [26, 48, 60–63]. Identifying changes in bacterial virulence production has highlighted an important role of bacterial toxin production causing increased host tissue damage during these infections. Furthermore, these efforts have led to a more complete understanding of the mechanisms influencing susceptibility and severity of secondary bacterial pneumonia, as they not only consider the contributions of the viral infection on host immunity, but account for the contributions of the host and virus towards the pathogenesis of bacterial species.

Commensals of the anterior nares commonly grow in biofilm communities [64, 65]. Recent studies have demonstrated infection with influenza promotes biofilm dispersal and dissemination of *S. aureus* and *S. pneumoniae* into the LRT [60, 62]. Interestingly, in biofilm communities where both *S. aureus* and *S. pneumoniae* are present influenza induced dissemination was almost entirely restricted to *S. pneumoniae* [61]. This suggests interactions with influenza result in immediate transcriptional changes that trigger *S. pneumoniae* biofilm dispersal while simultaneously suppressing *S. aureus* biofilm dispersal [61]. In addition, influenza can directly interact with surface of Gram-positive and Gram-negative organisms [66]. Virus bound to the surface of *S. aureus*, *S. pneumoniae*, and *H. influenzae* has been demonstrated to enhance bacterial adherence to epithelial cells [66].

One of the primary environmental factors that effects *S. pneumoniae* virulence is nutrition availability [57]. Carbohydrates are a necessary carbon source for pneumococcal growth [67]. Destruction of the epithelia tissue due to viral replication leads to increased mucus accumulation and decreased mucociliary clearance [21]. The accumulation of carbohydrate-rich mucus in the LRT promotes *S. pneumoniae* growth and production of epithelial adherence proteins [57, 62]. Intrinsic *S. pneumoniae* neuraminidase activity in combination with influenza neuraminidase activity during viral exit, desialylate the surface of host cells providing an additional carbohydrate source in the form of sialic acid [68, 69]. Continuous viral replication induces reactive oxygen species (ROS) generation from host cells. The presence of viral-induced ROS leads to an upregulation of the *S. pneumoniae* cytotoxin pneumolysin and causes enhanced necroptosis of the lung epithelium [70]. Taken together, these observations demonstrate a synergistic effect of *S. pneumoniae* growth and virulence with influenza infection.

There is substantial overlap regarding the broad effects of influenza infection on *S. pneumoniae* and *S. aureus*. Both organisms demonstrated enhanced dissemination into the lungs and upregulation of virulence genes during influenza infection [26, 61, 62, 70]. Evidence suggests that immediately upon being trafficked into the LRT, *S. aureus* forms microaggregates in the crypts of the alveolar wall [71]. These microaggregates secrete alpha-hemolysin (Hla), a toxin described to effect human alveolar macrophages and promote lung damage [72–74]. Gene regulation of *hla* is predominantly controlled by the two-component regulatory system SaeR/S and protein expression through the global gene regulator Agr [75, 76]. Agr regulates expression through quorum sensing and may be playing a role in Hla during microaggregate growth [75]. In a murine model of secondary *S. aureus* pneumonia, influenza infected mice demonstrated immediate upregulation of the *S. aureus* genes *saeR* and *saeS* and *saeR/S*-regulated toxins over mock infected mice [26]. Furthermore, mice challenged with a *saeR/S* isogenic gene deletion mutant strain of *S. aureus* displayed 100% survival compared to only 30% survival in mice challenged with wild-type *S. aureus* [26]. These data clearly demonstrate that the contributions of the bacterial pathogen towards *S. aureus* secondary bacterial pneumonia morbidity and mortality are, at minimum, of equal importance to the effects of influenza infection on host immune defenses.

3. Conclusion

A disease that has paralleled human progress throughout history is now just beginning to be understood. It is now apparent that the contributions to the increased susceptibility, morbidity, and mortality associated with secondary bacterial pneumonia following influenza infection span multiple disciplines (**Figure 1**). Undoubtedly, the effects of an influenza infection on the host immune system play a substantial role in increasing susceptibility to bacterial infection. Tissue damage, dysregulation of cytokine signaling, and suppression of phagocyte activity create an environmental niche primed for bacterial exploitation. However, more recent data have demonstrated changes in innate immune function alone are incomplete towards defining how bacteria transition from commensals to pathogens. This has prompted studies examining the ability of bacteria to sense and respond to the changes induced during and after influenza infection. Findings have demonstrated viral infection directly impacts bacterial pathogenesis by increasing bacterial dissemination, binding to epithelia, and upregulating virulence production. Taken together, these data indicate that a more thorough understanding necessitates additional studies to interrogate the contribution of host, viral, and bacterial interactions towards secondary bacterial pneumonia following influenza infection.

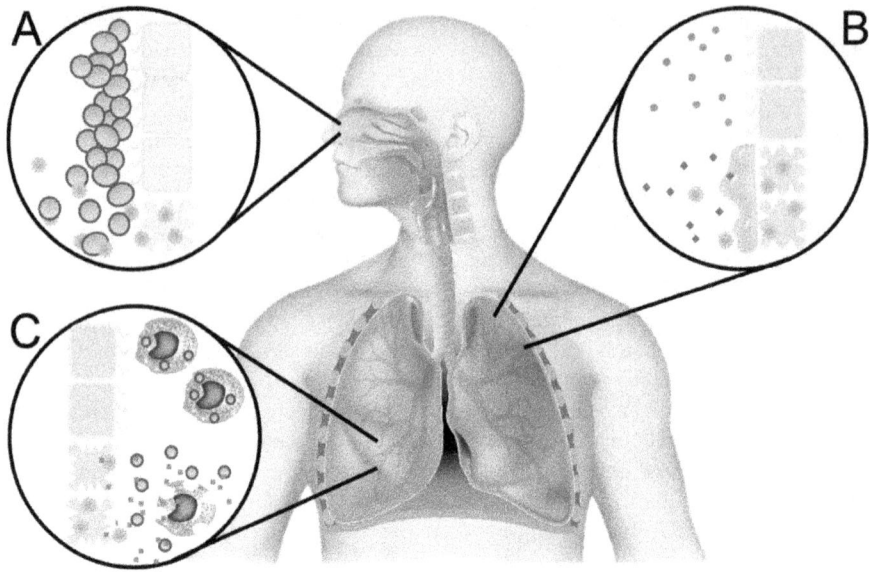

Figure 1.
Influenza infection enhances secondary bacterial pneumonia. (A) Increased dissemination into the LRT, (B) dysregulation of cytokine production and mucus accumulation, and (C) toxin production and tissue damage and reduced phagocytic function.

Acknowledgements

This work was supported by grants U54GM115371 and RO1AI149491 from the National Institutes of Health, and Montana State University Agriculture Experiment Station.

Conflict of interest

The authors declare no conflict of interest.

Declarations

Portions of this chapter were adapted from Borgogna T. Initiation and Pathogenesis of *Staphylococcus aureus* Pneumonia following Influenza A Infection [Dissertation]. Montana State University; 2019.

Author details

Timothy R. Borgogna* and Jovanka M. Voyich
Montana State University, Bozeman, MT, United States of America

*Address all correspondence to: timothy.borgogna@montana.edu

IntechOpen

References

[1] Gerdil C. The annual production cycle for influenza vaccine. Vaccine. 2003;**21**(16):1776-1779

[2] Potter CW. A history of influenza. Journal of Applied Microbiology. 2001;**91**(4):572-579. DOI: 10.1046/j.1365-2672.2001.01492.x

[3] Lina B. History of Influenza Pandemics. In: Raoult D, Drancourt M, editors. Paleomicrobiology. Berlin, Heidelberg: Springer; 2008. ISBN:978-3-540-75854-9 Online ISBN: 978-3-540-75855-6. DOI: 10.1007/978-3-540-75855-6_12

[4] Ashley WJ, Creighton C. A history of epidemics in Britain, from A.D. 664 to the extinction of plague. Political Science Quarterly. 1892;7(3):375-413

[5] Cornaglia G, Raoult D. Sometimes they come back-the return of influenza. Clinical Microbiology and Infection. 2011;**17**(5):647-648

[6] Muñoz-Sanz A. Christopher Columbus flu. A hypothesis for an ecological catastrophe. Enfermedades Infecciosas y Microbiología Clínica. 2006;**24**(5):236-334

[7] Guerra F. The earliest American epidemic. The influenza of 1493. Social Science History. 1988;**12**(3):305-325

[8] Curtin PD, Patterson KD. Pandemic influenza, 1700-1900: A study in historical epidemiology. The American Historical Review. 1988;**93**(3):1-118

[9] Spreeuwenberg P, Kroneman M, Paget J. Reassessing the global mortality burden of the 1918 influenza pandemic. American Journal of Epidemiology. 2018;**187**(12):2561-2567. DOI: 10.1093/aje/kwy191

[10] Grist NR. Pandemic influenza 1918. British Medical Journal. 1979;**2**(6205):1632-1633

[11] Morens DM, Taubenberger JK, Fauci AS. Predominant role of bacterial pneumonia as a cause of death in pandemic influenza: Implications for pandemic influenza preparedness. The Journal of Infectious Diseases. 2008;**198**(7):962-970

[12] Van Epps HL. Influenza: Exposing the true killer. Journal of Experimental Medicine. 2006;**203**(4):803

[13] Olitsky PK, Gates FL. Experimental studies of the nasopharyngeal secretions from influenza patients: Filterability and resistance to glycerol. The Journal of Experimental Medicine. 1921;**33**(3):361-372

[14] Shope RE. Swine influenza: III. Filtration experiments and etiology. Journal of Experimental Medicine. 1931;**54**(3):373-385

[15] Lewis PA, Shope RE. Swine influenza: II. A hemophilic bacillus from the respiratory tract of infected swine. The Journal of Experimental Medicine. 1931;**54**(3):361-371

[16] Paget J et al. "Global mortality associated with seasonal influenza epidemics: New burden estimates and predictors from the GLaMOR Project." Journal of global health. 2019;**9**(2):020421. DOI: 10.7189/jogh.09.020421

[17] Paget J, Spreeuwenberg P, Charu V, et al. Global mortality associated with seasonal influenza epidemics: New burden estimates and predictors from the GLaMOR project. Journal of Global Health. 2019;**9**(2):20421

[18] Lafond KE, Porter RM, Whaley MJ, et al. Global burden of influenza-associated lower respiratory tract infections and hospitalizations among adults: A systematic review and meta-analysis. PLoS Medicine. 2021;**18**(3):e1003550

[19] Rothberg MB, Haessler SD, Brown RB. Complications of viral influenza. The American Journal of Medicine. 2008;**121**(4):258-264

[20] Smetana J, Chlibek R, Shaw J, Splino M, Prymula R. Influenza vaccination in the elderly. Human Vaccines & Immunotherapeutics. 2018;**14**(3):540-549

[21] Hanada S, Pirzadeh M, Carver KY, Deng JC. Respiratory viral infection-induced microbiome alterations and secondary bacterial pneumonia. Frontiers in Immunology. 2018;**9**:2640. DOI: 10.3389/fimmu.2018.02640

[22] Morris DE, Cleary DW, Clarke SC. Secondary bacterial infections associated with influenza pandemics. Frontiers in Microbiology. 2017;**8**:1041

[23] Murphy SL, Xu J, Kochanek KD, Arias E, Tejada-Vera B. Deaths: Final data for 2018. National Vital Statistics Reports. 2021;**69**(13):24

[24] Kochanek KD, Murphy SL, Xu J, Arias E. Deaths: Final data for 2017. National Vital Statistics Reports. 2019;**68**(9):30

[25] Xu J, Murphy S, Kochanek K, Arias E. Deaths: Final data for 2019. National Vital Statistics Reports. 2021;**70**(8):25

[26] Borgogna TR, Hisey B, Heitmann E, Obar JJ, Meissner N, Voyich JM. Secondary bacterial pneumonia by *Staphylococcus aureus* following influenza A infection is SaeR/S dependent. Journal of Infectious Diseases. 2018;**218**(5):809-813

[27] Papanicolaou GA. Severe influenza and *S. aureus* pneumonia for whom the bell tolls? Virulence. 2013;**4**(8):666-668

[28] McCullers JA. The co-pathogenesis of influenza viruses with bacteria in the lung. Nature Reviews Microbiology. 2014;**12**:252-262

[29] Alymova IV, McCullers JA, Kamal RP, et al. Virulent PB1-F2 residues: Effects on fitness of H1N1 influenza A virus in mice and changes during evolution of human influenza A viruses. Scientific Reports. 2018;**8**:7474. DOI: 10.1038/s41598-018-25707-y

[30] Iverson AR, Boyd KL, McAuley JL, Plano LR, Hart ME, McCullers JA. Influenza virus primes mice for pneumonia from *Staphylococcus aureus*. The Journal of Infectious Diseases. 2011;**203**(6):880-888. DOI: 10.1093/infdis/jiq113

[31] McAuley JL, Hornung F, Boyd KL, et al. Expression of the 1918 influenza A virus PB1-F2 enhances the pathogenesis of viral and secondary bacterial pneumonia. Cell Host & Microbe. 2007;**2**(4):240-249

[32] Louria DB, Blumenfeld HL, Ellis JT, Kilbourne ED, Rogers DE. Studies on influenza in the pandemic of 1957-1958. II. Pulmonary complications of influenza. The Journal of Clinical Investigation. 1959;**38**(1 Part 2):213-265

[33] Lee MH, Arrecubieta C, Martin FJ, Prince A, Borczuk AC, Lowy FD. A postinfluenza model of *Staphylococcus aureus* pneumonia. Journal of Infectious Diseases. 2010;**201**(4):508-515

[34] Wilden JJ, Jacob JC, Ehrhardt C, Ludwig S, Boergeling Y. Altered signal transduction in the immune response to influenza virus and *S. pneumoniae* or *S. aureus* co-infections. International Journal of Molecular Sciences. 2021;**22**(11):5486

[35] Gorwitz RJ, Kruszon-Moran D, McAllister SK, et al. Changes in the prevalence of nasal colonization with *Staphylococcus aureus* in the United States, 2001-2004. Journal of Infectious Diseases. 2008;**197**(9):1226-1234

[36] Sender V, Hentrich K, Henriques-Normark B. Virus-induced changes of the respiratory tract environment promote secondary infections with *Streptococcus pneumoniae*. Frontiers in Cellular and Infection Microbiology. 2021;**11**: 643326

[37] Tufvesson E, Markstad H, Bozovic G, Ekberg M, Bjermer L. Inflammation and chronic colonization of *Haemophilus influenzae* in sputum in COPD patients related to the degree of emphysema and bronchiectasis in high-resolution computed tomography. International Journal of Chronic Obstructive Pulmonary Disease. 2017; **12**:3211-3219

[38] Herrera AL, Huber VC, Chaussee MS. The association between invasive group A streptococcal diseases and viral respiratory tract infections. Frontiers in Microbiology. 2016;**7**:342

[39] Klonoski JM, Watson T, Bickett TE, et al. Contributions of influenza virus hemagglutinin and host immune responses toward the severity of influenza virus: *Streptococcus pyogenes* superinfections. Viral Immunology. 2018;**31**(6):457-469

[40] Huffnagle GB, Dickson RP. The bacterial microbiota in inflammatory lung diseases. Clinical Immunology. 2015;**159**(2):177-182

[41] Dickson RP, Erb-Downward JR, Martinez FJ, Huffnagle GB. The microbiome and the respiratory tract. Annual Review of Physiology. 2016;**78**:481-504

[42] van der Sluijs KF, van der Poll T, Lutter R, Juffermans NP, Schultz MJ. Bench-to-bedside review: Bacterial pneumonia with influenza— Pathogenesis and clinical implications. Critical Care. 2010;**14**(2):219

[43] Iwasaki A, Pillai PS. Innate immunity to influenza virus infection.

Nature Reviews Immunology. 2014;**14**(5):315-328

[44] Robinson KM, Kolls JK, Alcorn JF. The immunology of influenza virus-associated bacterial pneumonia. Current Opinion in Immunology. 2015;**34**:59-67

[45] Plotkowski MC, Puchelle E, Beck G, Jacquot J, Hannoun C. Adherence of type I *Streptococcus pneumoniae* to tracheal epithelium of mice infected with influenza A/PR8 virus. American Review of Respiratory Disease. 1986;**134**(5):1040-1044

[46] Rynda-Apple A, Robinson KM, Alcorn JF. Influenza and bacterial superinfection: Illuminating the immunologic mechanisms of disease. Infection and Immunity. 2015;**83**(10):3764-3770

[47] Ghoneim HE, Thomas PG, McCullers JA. Depletion of alveolar macrophages during influenza infection facilitates bacterial superinfections. The Journal of Immunology. 2013;**191**(3):1250-1259

[48] Verma AK, Bansal S, Bauer C, Muralidharan A, Sun K. Influenza infection induces alveolar macrophage dysfunction and thereby enables noninvasive *Streptococcus pneumoniae* to cause deadly pneumonia. The Journal of Immunology. 2020;**205**(6):1601-1607

[49] Abramson JS, Mills EL, Giebink GS, Quie PG. Depression of monocyte and polymorphonuclear leukocyte oxidative metabolism and bactericidal capacity by influenza A virus. Infection and Immunity. 1982;**35**(1):350-355

[50] Camp JV, Jonsson CB. A role for neutrophils in viral respiratory disease. Frontiers in Immunology. 2017:**8**

[51] Smith AM, Adler FR, Ribeiro RM, et al. Kinetics of coinfection with influenza A virus and *Streptococcus*

pneumoniae. PLoS Pathogens. 2013;**9**(3):e1003238. DOI: 10.1371/journal.ppat.1003238

[52] Laichalk LL, Danforth JM, Standiford TJ. Interleukin-10 inhibits neutrophil phagocytic and bactericidal activity. FEMS Immunology and Medical Microbiology. 1996;**15**(4):181-187

[53] Kudva A, Scheller EV, Robinson KM, et al. Influenza A inhibits Th17-mediated host defense against bacterial pneumonia in mice. The Journal of Immunology. 2011;**186**(3):1666-1674

[54] Robinson KM, McHugh KJ, Mandalapu S, et al. Influenza A virus exacerbates *Staphylococcus aureus* pneumonia in mice by attenuating antimicrobial peptide production. Journal of Infectious Diseases. 2014;**209**(6):865-875

[55] Shepardson KM, Larson K, Morton RV, et al. Differential type I interferon signaling is a master regulator of susceptibility to postinfluenza bacterial superinfection. MBio. 2016;7(3)

[56] Subramaniam R, Barnes PF, Fletcher K, et al. Protecting against post-influenza bacterial pneumonia by increasing phagocyte recruitment and ROS production. Journal of Infectious Diseases. 2014;**209**(11):1827-1836

[57] Sun K, Metzger DW. Influenza infection suppresses NADPH oxidase-dependent phagocytic bacterial clearance and enhances susceptibility to secondary methicillin-resistant *Staphylococcus aureus* infection. The Journal of Immunology. 2014;**192**(7):3301-3307

[58] Karwelat D, Schmeck B, Ringel M, et al. Influenza virus-mediated suppression of bronchial Chitinase-3-like 1 secretion promotes secondary pneumococcal infection. FASEB Journal. 2020;**34**(12):16432-16448

[59] Metzger DW, Sun K. Immune dysfunction and bacterial coinfections following influenza. The Journal of Immunology. 2013;**191**(5):2047

[60] Reddinger RM, Luke-Marshall NR, Hakansson AP, Campagnari AA. Host physiologic changes induced by influenza a virus lead to *Staphylococcus aureus* biofilm dispersion and transition from asymptomatic colonization to invasive disease. MBio. 2016;**7**(4)

[61] Reddinger RM, Luke-Marshall NR, Sauberan SL, Hakansson AP, Campagnari AA. *Streptococcus pneumoniae* modulates *Staphylococcus aureus* biofilm dispersion and the transition from colonization to invasive disease. MBio. 2018;**9**(1)

[62] Pettigrew MM, Marks LR, Kong Y, Gent JF, Roche-Hakansson H, Hakansson AP. Dynamic changes in the *Streptococcus pneumoniae* transcriptome during transition from biofilm formation to invasive disease upon influenza A virus infection. Infection and Immunity. 2014;**82**(11):4607-4619

[63] Borgogna TR, Sanchez-Gonzalez A, Gorham K, Voyich JM. A precise pathogen delivery and recovery system for murine models of secondary bacterial pneumonia. Journal of Visualized Experiments. 2019;**2019**(151)

[64] Scherr TD, Heim CE, Morrison JM, Kielian T. Hiding in plain sight: Interplay between staphylococcal biofilms and host immunity. Frontiers in Immunology. 2014;**5**

[65] Kumpitsch C, Koskinen K, Schöpf V, Moissl-Eichinger C. The microbiome of the upper respiratory tract in health and disease. BMC Biology. 2019;**17**

[66] Rowe HM, Meliopoulos VA, Iverson A, Bomme P, Schultz-Cherry S, Rosch JW. Direct interactions with influenza promote bacterial adherence

during respiratory infections. Nature Microbiology. 2019;**4**(8):1328-1336

[67] Buckwalter CM, King SJ. Pneumococcal carbohydrate transport: Food for thought. Trends in Microbiology. 2012;**20**(11):517-522

[68] Siegel SJ, Roche AM, Weiser JN. Influenza promotes pneumococcal growth during coinfection by providing host sialylated substrates as a nutrient source. Cell Host & Microbe. 2014;**16**(1):55-67

[69] du Toit A. Pneumococci find a sugar daddy in influenza. Nature Reviews Microbiology. 2014;**12**(9):596

[70] Gonzalez-Juarbe N, Riegler AN, Jureka AS, et al. Influenza-induced oxidative stress sensitizes lung cells to bacterial-toxin-mediated necroptosis. Cell Reports. 2020;**32**(8)

[71] Hook JL, Islam MN, Parker D, Prince AS, Bhattacharya S, Bhattacharya J. Disruption of staphylococcal aggregation protects against lethal lung injury. Journal of Clinical Investigation. 2018;**128**(3):1074-1086

[72] Brann KR, Fullerton MS, Onyilagha FI, et al. Infection of primary human alveolar macrophages alters *Staphylococcus aureus* toxin production and activity. Infection and Immunity. 2019;**87**(7)

[73] Parker D, Prince A. Immunopathogenesis of *Staphylococcus aureus* pulmonary infection. Seminars in Immunopathology. 2012;**34**(2):281-297

[74] Kitur K, Parker D, Nieto P, et al. Toxin-induced necroptosis is a major mechanism of *Staphylococcus aureus* lung damage. PLoS Pathogens. 2015;**11**(4)

[75] Jenul C, Horswill AR. Regulation of *Staphylococcus aureus* virulence. Microbiology Spectrum. 2019;**7**(2)

[76] Flack CE, Zurek OW, Meishery DD, et al. Differential regulation of staphylococcal virulence by the sensor kinase SaeS in response to neutrophil-derived stimuli. Proceedings of the National Academy of Sciences of the United States of America. 2014;**111**(19):2037-2045

Chapter 5

Proteins of *Streptococcus pneumoniae* Involved in Iron Acquisition

José de Jesús Olivares-Trejo
and María Elizbeth Alvarez-Sánchez

Abstract

Streptococcus pneumoniae is a human pathogen bacterium capable of using hemoglobin (Hb) and haem as a single iron source but not in presence of lactoferrin. This bacterium has developed a mechanism through the expression of several membrane proteins that bind to iron sources, between them a lipoprotein of 37 kDa called Spbhp-37 (*Streptococcus pneumoniae* haem-binding protein) involved in iron acquisition. The Spbhp-37 role is to maintain the viability of *S. pneumoniae* in presence of Hb or haem. This mechanism is relevant during the invasion of *S. pneumoniae* to human tissue for the acquisition of iron from hemoglobin or haem as an iron source.

Keywords: *S. pneumoniae*, haem, iron acquisition, hemoglobin, Hb-binding protein

1. Introduction

Iron is required for cellular growth of any bacterial species and it is known that bacterium needs an iron concentration of 10^{-6}–10^{-8} M [1, 2], however, the concentration of free iron in the human body is usually 10^{-18} M [3], lower than bacterial requirements [4–6]. Therefore, human pathogens often obtain iron from alternative sources available into the body such as lactoferrin (Holo-Lf), hemoglobin (Hb) or even the haem [7]. The success of pathogens to obtain iron from host sources is based on developing different mechanisms, for instance, a direct mechanism which consists of expressing proteins attach to the membrane (termed receptors) [8, 9].

Another mechanism (known as indirect mechanism) is based on secreting siderophores or haemophores to scavenge iron then it is delivering towards a receptor protein [10]. The transportation of iron into the cytoplasm requires proteins as the ATP-binding protein cassette (ABC) [11], these mechanisms have been established in Gram-negative but not in Gram-positive bacteria.

S. pneumoniae is a bacterium Gram-positive human pathogen, which causes otitis media, sinusitis, pneumonia, meningitis or bacteriemia especially in infants and elderly persons [12–16]. *S. pneumoniae* can grow under iron-restricted medium conditions, if the growth media is supplemented with ferric and ferrous iron salts, haem or Hb [17, 18], but not when Tf, Lf or ferritin (Ft) are added [19, 20]. Moreover, *S. pneumoniae* expresses the Spbhp-37 lipoprotein (37 KDa) on its surface, which binds both haem and Hb. Spbhp-37 lipoprotein binds its ligand with high affinity because has a Kd of 3.57 e-7 M [21]. The interaction between

Sphbp-37 lipoprotein can be inhibited with antibodies specific against this lipo-protein. These findings furthermore suggest that this lipoprotein is a receptor protein attached to the membrane of *S. pneumoniae* that binds haem. Despite these findings, the interaction molecular between Sphbp-37 lipoprotein and haem has not been analyzed yet and neither how *spbhp-37* gene expression occurs when haem binds to the lipoprotein. To dilucidated how the lipoprotein binds haem a strategy could be designed, for instance, investigate 3D structure, the interaction between the Sphbp-37 lipoprotein and haem, or amino acid residues that interact with haem and levels of mRNA of the *spbhp-37*. The aim of this chapter attempt to explain how *S. pneumoniae* binds the iron source and the pathway developed to increase its levels of iron maybe this increase help to this pathogen to invade multiple human tissues, in the future this information could be utilized to develop new treatment allowing better control of this human pathogen.

2. *S. pneumoniae* iron acquisition

S. pneumoniae has the polysaccharide capsule and various virulence factors of *S. pneumoniae* that participate in its pathogenesis and facilitate its dissemination [22]. As any bacterium needs iron for several essential functions like the electron transport chain, energy metabolism, and many other biological functions [23], this element can be obtained from human sources such as hemoglobin (Hb), haem (from erythrocytes) ferritin (from serum and secretions) and glycoproteins (transferrin and lactoferrin) [24, 25]. Interestingly *S. pneumoniae* proteome does not have ferritin binding proteins (FBPs) [26] and also lacks of siderophores [27] because the large layer of the capsule avoids the presence of siderophores binding protein. To obtain iron for sources like ferritin, this pathogen has developed a smart mechanism that consists on to express PspA protein, this protein plays a key role in binding to lactoferrin at the pneumococ-cal surface. This mechanism could be useful in tissues like epithelial secretions where lactoferrin is the only source of iron. The expression of PspA is associated with the reduced concentration of free iron in secretions [28]. In vitro studies have showed that, the concentration of ferritin can be preserved in the culture media when a pro-tease inhibitor (PMSF) is added, also molecular docking of pneumococcal proteases such as HtrA, ClpP, and RadA has revealed that those proteases could be inhibited by the PMSF [26]. Therefore, these observations indicated that *S. pneumoniae* may recruit protease-dependent pathways to obtain iron. Such pathways provide several effective strategies obviating the need for specific receptors and transporters.

3. Hb-binding proteins involved in iron acquisition

Iron is also available in human sources for instance hemoglobin or haem structure within erythrocytes. *S. pneumoniae* expressed and secreted an Hb and haem-binding protein of 38 kDa. This protein has a multitasking function because was identified by mass spectrometry as glyceraldehyde-3-phosphate dehydrogenase (GAPDH) a protein involved in metabolism principally. *S. pneumoniae* secretes GAPDH and this is protein is capable of binding two useful iron sources for this bacterium (Hb and haem). This protein could be playing a dynamic role in the success of the invasive and infective processes of this pathogen [29]. Additionally, *S. pneumoniae* is a pathogen capable of supporting its viability when iron sources such as Hb or haem are supplied. This bacterium can express two haem and Hb-binding proteins on its cytoplasmic membrane, whose molecular weights are 37 and 22 kDa respectively. Their respective names are Spbhp-37 and Spbhp-22 (*S. pneumoniae* Hb- and haem-binding proteins

37 and 22 kDa). The Hb-binding function in both proteins has been demonstrated using Hb and the respective identities of both proteins have been obtained by mass spectrometry. The amino acid sequences of both Hb-binding proteins have the motif involved in the binding of Hb or haem. Specifically, Spbhp-37 protein is founded in the surface of this pathogen. The expression of Spbhp-37 is increased when the bacterium is grown in media culture supplied with Hb this finding corroborates the importance of this protein in the Hb-binding. It could explain the mechanisms developed by *S. pneumoniae* to acquire iron from Hb or haem in the host, which could allow a better understanding of the biology of this bacterium.

4. Hb-iron transporters

The necessity to obtain iron in the human host has provided *S. pneumoniae* with a sophisticated mechanism. PiaA is a hemoglobin-binding protein localized on the surface of *S. pneumoniae* [27]. Moreover, Pit, Pia, and Piu have emerged as other possible iron transporters of *S. pneumoniae* [28]. Brown et al. reported that ABC transporter-like proteins, may be involved in iron absorption by *S. pneumoniae* [19, 20]. Overall, all these proteins further participate in the acquisition of this essential metal for the survival of this pathogen.

5. Which are the amino acid residues of Sphbp-37 haem-binding protein involved in the interaction with the iron source?

5.1 3D modeling of Sphbp-37 protein

To understand more about the interaction between haem-binding protein Sphbp-37 and iron source an *in silico* approach can be performed, for instance, 3D modeling of Sphbp-37 protein shows a globular structure (**Figure 1A**). This structure has nine α-helices and eleven β-sheet. After molecular dynamic simulation of 500 ns by I-TASSER server, Sphbp-37 protein stills its globular structure, showing the same number of α-helices, although the number of β-sheet was increased to thirteen (**Figure 1B**). Therefore the analysis of time-dependent motions of the Sphbp-37 protein by RMSD shows that this molecule gets its equilibrium after 500 ns (**Figure 2A**). Rg values show the protein expansion after 100 and 200 ns and a compactation at the last 20 ns (**Figure 2B**). RMSF value show a moderate fluctuation in some amino acid (**Figure 2C**).

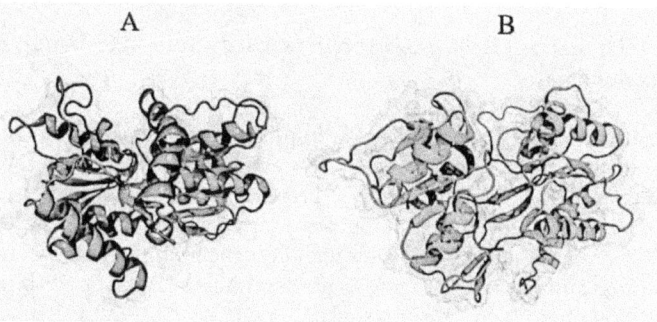

Figure 1.
3D Modeling of Sphbp-37 protein before (A) and after (B) of 500 ns dynamic molecular simulation by I-TASSER program.

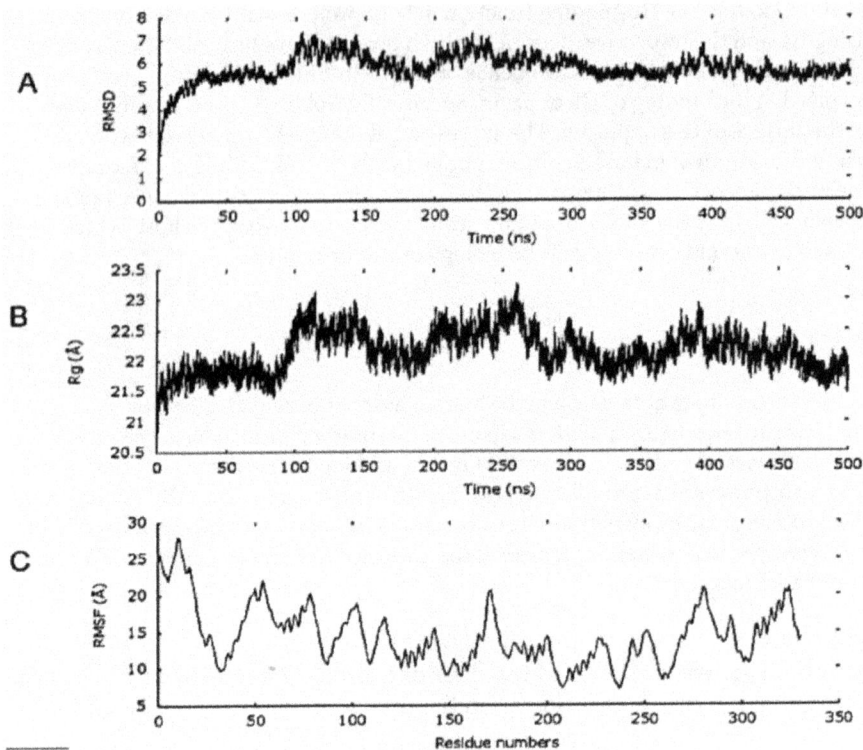

Figure 2.
RMSD analysis of Sphbp-37 protein (A). Rg values show the protein expansion after 100 and 200 ns and a compactation at the last 20 ns (B). RMSF values (C).

5.2 Interaction of Sphbp-37 protein with haem

We search the amino acids involved in the between Sphbp-37 protein and haem. The molecular dynamic simulation after 500 ns shows an interaction between haem and amino acid residues of Sphbp-37 protein: glutamic acid 152 (Glu152), glutamine 177 (Gln177), valine 178 (Val178), aspartic acid 179 (Asp179), tyrosine 180 (Tyr180), isoleucine 193 (Ile193), alanine 196 (Ala196), glutamine 197 (Gln197) and alanine 200 (Ala200) (**Figure 3**). We found 10 amino acids involved in the interaction of Sphbp-37 and haem.

5.3 3D model of mutant Sphbp-37 protein (substitutions in 152 and 179 amino acid residues)

To investigate which amino acids of Sphbp-37 protein are involved in haem-binding, we performed a change of glu152 for alanine (glu152ala) and asp179 for alanine ala (asp179ala) (mutant Sphbp-37 protein), these amino acid directly binds the haem. The result showed that the substitution of amino acid in the position 152 and 179 by another amino acid does not allow the binding to the haem. These data shown that amino acids 152 and 179 are essential for haem or Hb-binding and participate direct binding of the iron source.

3D model of mutant Sphbp-37 protein with changes in 152 and 179 amino acid residues was analyzed by NAMD software, the result showed a globular structure inclusive after the changes, however, the binding is not preserved (**Figure 4**).

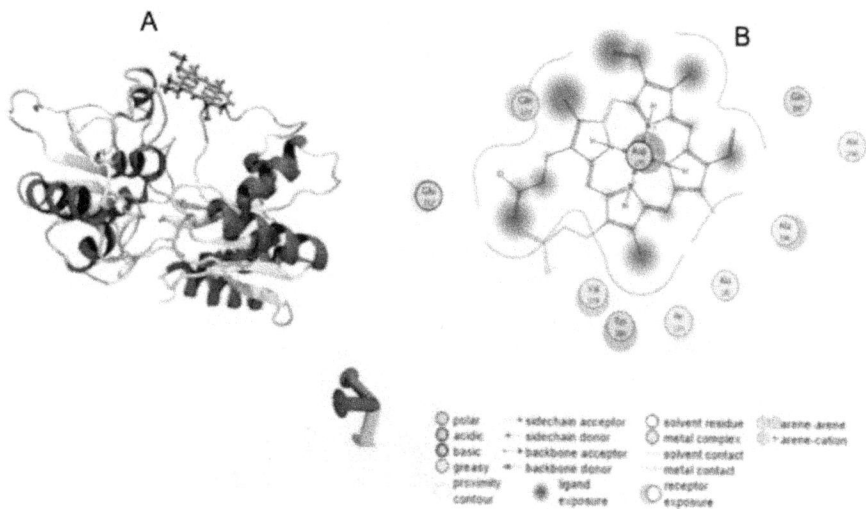

Figure 3.
Molecular analysis between Sphbp-37 lipoprotein and haem. (A) Interaction between Sphbp-37 lipoprotein and haem. (B) The 10 amino acid residues, which are showed in green and pink color.

Mutant Sphbp-37 protein is unable to bind haem these results suggest that amino acids residues of 152 and 179 positions are involved in haem binding directly.

5.4 The promoter region of the spbhp-37 gene does not fur box consensus sequences

Then, we analyzed the *spbhp-37* gene and search a probable promoter sequence by the BPROM program. The analysis revealed the regions promoter −35 and −10 located upstream from the start codon (**Figure 5A**). The promoter sequence of the *spbhp-37* gene does not align with the consensus Fur box of *E. coli* [30] and other Fur box-like sequences previously reported such as *dhb* [31], *fhu* [32] the *fhu* and *sir* operons from *B. subtilis* [33] and operons from *S. aureus*, with the program Jalview (http://www.jalview.org). The alignment showed a different sequence from those previously reported, showing only a 26% of identity when the sequence promoter of *S.*

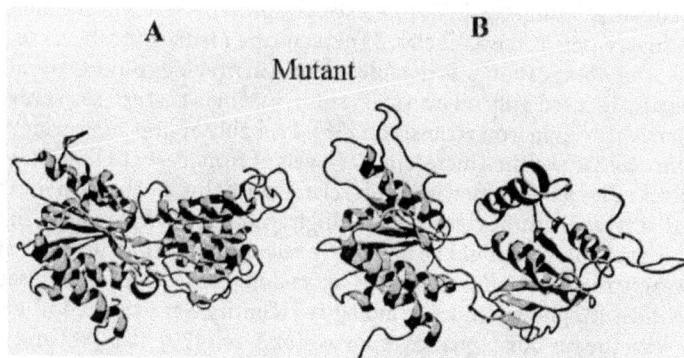

Figure 4.
3D modeling of Sphbp-37 mutant before (A) and after (B) of 500 ns of molecular dynamic simulation by I-TASSER server. Amino acid residues of 152 position (glu) and 179 position (asp) were substituted by the ala. The globular structure was maintained.

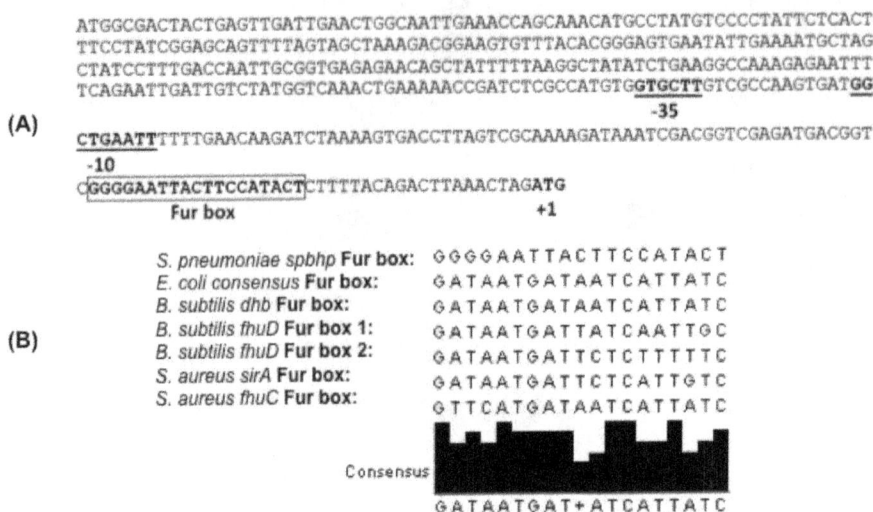

```
ATGGCGACTACTGAGTTGATTGAACTGGCAATTGAAACCAGCAAACATGCCTATGTCCCCTATTCTCACT
TTCCTATCGGAGCAGTTTTAGTAGCTAAAGACGGAAGTGTTTACACGGGAGTGAATATTGAAAATGCTAG
CTATCCTTTGACCAATTGCGGTGAGAGAACAGCTATTTTTAAGGCTATATCTGAAGGCCAAAGAGAATTT
TCAGAATTGATTGTCTATGGTCAAACTGAAAAACCGATCTCGCCATGTGGTGCTTGTCGCCAAGTGATGG
                                                        -35
CTGAATTTTTTGAACAAGATCTAAAAGTGACCTTAGTCGCAAAAGATAAATCGACGGTCGAGATGACGGT
 -10
CGGGGAATTACTTCCATACTCTTTTACAGACTTAAACTAGAATG
    Fur box                              +1
```

(A)

(B)

S. pneumoniae spbhp **Fur box:**	G G G G A A T T A C T T C C A T A C T
E. coli consensus **Fur box:**	G A T A A T G A T A A T C A T T A T C
B. subtilis dhb **Fur box:**	G A T A A T G A T A A T C A T T A T C
B. subtilis fhuD **Fur box 1:**	G A T A A T G A T T A T C A A T T G C
B. subtilis fhuD **Fur box 2:**	G A T A A T G A T T C T C T T T T T C
S. aureus sirA **Fur box:**	G A T A A T G A T T C T C A T T G T C
S. aureus fhuC **Fur box:**	G T T C A T G A T A A T C A T T A T C

Consensus

G A T A A T G A T + A T C A T T A T C

Figure 5.
Promoter predicted elements for spbhp-37 gene. (A) Schematic organization of spbhp-37 promoter, the translation-initiation codon ATG +1, −35 and − 10 regions of the promoter sequence are indicated in bold type and underlined. The box indicates the conserved fur-binding sequences. (B) Alignment of the consensus "fur box" sequences of E. coli, dhb and fhu of B. subtilis, fhu and sir of S. aureus and the spbhp-37. The differences are indicated in the boxes.

pneumoniae is compared with the consensus fur-box sequence of *E. coli* (**Figure 5B**). This analysis suggests that the promoter sequence of *S. pneumoniae* does not have *fur-box* and perhaps the regulation could be by a different mechanism (data in progress).

6. Discussion

S. pneumoniae is a pathogen that uses Hb and haem as only iron sources. It also expresses a lipoprotein Sphbp-37 that participates in iron acquisition binding Hb and haem [17]. This chapter presents the first effort to understand how *S. pneumoniae* can be stimulated for iron acquisition: under iron starvation, which could occur as in other bacterial pathogens such as *Vibrio sp.*, *Pseudomonas aeruginosa*, *Escherichia coli*, *Shigella flexneri*, *Bacillus subtilis* [34] or with Holo-Tf stimulation such as occurs in *E. histolytica* [35]. Interestingly, proteins levels of the Sphbp-37 increased: first, when iron was chelated from culture media and Hb was used as an iron source, this observation was notable because in previous reports the attention was principally focused only on iron starvation, in which there is an overexpression of genes participating in iron acquisition [36]. Probably Sphbp-37 is overexpressed when *S. pneumoniae* requires increasing its levels of iron. Perhaps the whole mechanism involves other genes which have not related with this mechanism for instance *hemolysin* that lyses erythrocytes to release high amounts of Hb or haem, in this manner, it is available and could be use by *S. pneumoniae*. *In silico* analysis of 200 nucleotides upstream from the *sphbp-37* start codon revealed a promoter sequence with nucleotides [37] however, no homology or identity was observed when it was compared with the fur box sequence reported for *E. coli* [30], *dhb* [31] and *fhu* [32]), operons of *B. subtilis*, the *fhu* and *sir* [33] and operons of *S. aureus*. This data suggests that the differences observed in the nucleotide sequences could be related with a regulation mechanism of *S. pneumoniae* that involves many proteins, but different to described for Gram-negative bacteria [38]. Maybe all these proteins are involved in the binding to iron, haem or Hb-binding proteins and are necessary when the pathogen invades tissue. Finally, it does not discard the possibility that this type of regulation occurs in other bacterial pathogens.

Conflict of interest

The authors declare that they have no conflict of interest.

Author details

José de Jesús Olivares-Trejo* and María Elizbeth Alvarez-Sánchez
Posgrado en Ciencias Genómicas, Universidad Autónoma de la Ciudad de México, Mexico

*Address all correspondence to: olivarestrejo@yahoo.com

IntechOpen

References

[1] Ge R, Sun X. Iron trafficking system in *Helicobacter pylori*. Biometals. 2012;**25**:247-258

[2] Klebba PE, McIntosh MA, Neilands JB. Kinetics of biosynthesis of iron-regulated membrane proteins in *Escherichia coli*. Journal of Bacteriology. 1982;**149**:880-888

[3] Raymond KN, Dertz EA, Kim SS. Enterobactin: An archetype for microbial iron transport. Proceedings of the National Academy of Sciences. 2003;**100**:3584-3588

[4] Andrews S, Robinsón AK, Rodríguez-Quiñonez F. Bacterial iron homeostasis. FEMS Microbiology. 2003;**27**:215-237

[5] Horton R, Moran L, Ochs R, Rawn J, Scrimgeour K. Principles of Biochemistry. 3rd edition. Pearson; 2002. p. 827

[6] Ratledge C, Dover L. Iron metabolism in pathogenic bacteria. Annual Review of Microbiology. 2000;**54**:881-941

[7] Wooldridge KG, Williams PH. Iron uptake mechanisms of pathogenic bacteria. FEMS Microbiology. 1993;**12**: 325-348

[8] Guerinot ML. Microbial iron transport. Annual Review of Microbiology. 1994;**48**:743-772

[9] Wandersman C, Delepelaire P. Bacterial iron sources: From siderophores to haemophores. Annual Review of Microbiology. 2004;**58**:611-647

[10] Genco CA, Dixon DW. Emerging strategies in microbial haem capture. Molecular Microbiology. 2001;**39**:1-11

[11] Miethke M. Iron-responsive bacterial small RNAs: Variations on a theme. Metallomics. 2013;**5**:15-28

[12] Butler JC, Schuchat A. Epidemiology of pneumococcal infections in the elderly. Drugs & Aging. 1999;**15**:11-19

[13] Gray BM, Converse J, Dillon H. Serotypes of *Streptococcus pneumoniae* causing disease. The Journal of Infectious Diseases. 1979;**140**:979-983

[14] Musher DM. Infections caused by *Streptococcus pneumoniae*: Clinical spectrum, pathogenesis, immunity, and treatment. Clinical Infectious Diseases. 1992;**14**:801-807

[15] Thornton J, Durick-Eder K, Tuomanen E. Pneumococcal pathogenesis: "Innate invasion" yet organ-specific damage. Journal of Molecular Medicine. 2010;**88**:103-107

[16] Yaro S, Lourd M, Traoré Y, Njanpop-Lafourcade BM, Sawadogo A, Sangare L, et al. Epidemiological and molecular characteristics of a highly lethal pneumococcal meningitis epidemic in Burkina Faso. Clinical Infectious Diseases. 2006;**43**:693-700

[17] Romero-Espejel ME, González-López MA, Olivares-Trejo JJ. *Streptococcus pneumoniae* requires iron for its viability and expresses two membrane proteins that bind haemoglobin and haem. Metallomics. 2013;**5**:384-389

[18] Tai SS, Lee CJ, Winter RE. Hemin utilization is related to virulence of *Streptococcus pneumoniae*. *Infection* and *Immunity*. 1993;**61**:5401-5405

[19] Brown JS, Gilliland SM, Holden DW. A *Streptococcus pneumoniae* pathogenicity island encoding an ABC transporter involved in iron uptake and virulence. Molecular Microbiology. 2002;**40**:572-585

[20] Brown JS, Gilliland SM, Ruiz-Albert J, Holden DW. Characterization of pit, a *Streptococcus pneumoniae* iron uptake ABC

transporter. Infection and Immunity. 2002b;**70**(8):4389-4398. DOI: 10.1128/IAI.70.8.4389-4398

[21] Romero-Espejel ME, Rodríguez MA, Chávez-Munguía B, Ríos-Castro E, Olivares-Trejo JJ. Characterization of Spbhp-37, a Hemoglobin-binding protein of *Streptococcus pneumoniae*. Frontiers in Cellular and Infection Microbiology. 2016;**4**(6):47. DOI: 10.3389/fcimb..00047

[22] Yamamoto S, Shinoda S. Iron uptake mechanisms of pathogenic bacteria. Nihon Saikingaku Zasshi. 1996;**51**:523-547. DOI: 10.3412/jsb.51.523

[23] Cherayil BJ. The role of iron in the immune response to bacterial infection. Immunologic Research. 2011;**50**:1-9. DOI: 10.1007/s12026-010-8199-1

[24] Brock JH. The physiology of lactoferrin. Biochemistry and Cell Biology. 2002;**80**(1):1-6. DOI: 10.1139/o01-212

[25] Kawabata H, Sakamoto S, Masuda T. Roles of transferrin receptors in erythropoiesis. Rinsho Ketsueki The Japanese Journal of Clinical Hematology. 2016;**57**:951-958. DOI: 10.11406/rinketsu.57.951

[26] Kheirandish M, Motlagh B, Afshar D. Ferritin degradation by pneumococcal HtrA, RadA and ClpP serine proteases: A probable way for releasing and Acquisition of Iron. Infection and Drug Resistance. 2020;**13**:3145-3152. DOI: 10.2147/IDR.S264170

[27] Tai SS, Yu C, Lee JK. A solute binding protein of *Streptococcus pneumoniae* iron transport. FEMS Microbiology Letters. 2003;**220**:303-308. DOI: 10.1016/S0378-1097(03)00135-6

[28] Cheng W, Li Q, Jiang Y-L, Zhou C-Z, Chen Y. Structures of *Streptococcus pneumoniae* PiaA and its complex with ferrichrome reveal insights into the substrate binding and release of high

affinity iron transporters. PLoS One. 2013;**8**(8):e71451. DOI: 10.1371/journal.pone.0071451

[29] Vázquez-Zamorano ZE, González-López MA, Romero-Espejel ME, Azuara-Liceaga EI, López-Casamichana M, Olivares-Trejo JJ. *Streptococcus pneumoniae* secretes a glyceraldehyde-3-phosphate dehydrogenase, which binds haemoglobin and haem. Biometals. 2014;**27**:683-693. DOI: 10.1007/s10534-014-9757-0

[30] Lorenzo V, Giovannini F, Herrero M, Neilands JB. Metal ion regulation of gene expression: Fur repressor–operator interaction at the promoter region of the aerobactin system of pColV-K30. Journal of Molecular Biology. 1988;**203**:875-884

[31] Rowland BM, Grossman TH, Osburne MS, Taber HW. Sequence and genetic organization of a *Bacillus subtilis* operon encoding 2, 3-dihydroxybenzoate biosynthetic enzymes. Journal of Bacteriology. 1996;**178**:119-123

[32] Bsat N, Helmann JD. Interaction of *Bacillus subtilis* fur (ferric-uptake repressor) with the *dhb* operator in vitro and in vivo. Journal of Bacteriology. 1999;**181**:4299-4307

[33] Heinrich JH, Gatlin LE, Kunsch C, Choi GH, Hanson MS. Identification and characterization of SirA, an iron-regulated protein from *Staphylococcus aureus*. Journal of Bacteriology. 1999;**181**:1436-1443

[34] Masse E, Salvail H, Desnoyers G, Arguin M. Small RNAs controlling iron metabolism. Current Opinion in Microbiology. 2007;**10**:140-145

[35] Sánchez-Cruz C, López-Casamichana M, Cruz Castañeda A, Olivares-Trejo JJ. Transferrin regulates mRNA levels of a gene involved in iron utilization in *Entamoeba histolytica*. Molecular Biology Reports. 2011;**39**:4545-4551

[36] Gupta R, Shah P, Swiatlo E. Differential gene expression in *Streptococcus pneumoniae* in response to various iron sources. Microbial Pathogenesis. 2009;**47**:101-109

[37] Hoskins J, Alborn WE, Arnold J, Blaszczak LC, Burgett S, DeHoff BS, et al. Genome of the bacterium *Streptococcus pneumoniae* strain R6. Journal of Bacteriology. 2001;**183**:5709-5717

[38] Crosa J. Signal transduction and transcriptional and post-transcriptional control of iron-regulated genes in bacteria. Microbiology and Molecular Biology Reviews. 1997;**61**:319-336